Do-it-Yourself
HEALTH

D1367117

Do-it-Yourself HEALTH

1,001 TIPS YOU CAN USE TO FEEL BETTER AND STAY WELL

by the Editors of Time-Life Books
Alexandria, Virginia

Do-it-Yourself
HEALTH

**TIME-LIFE BOOKS IS A
DIVISION OF TIME LIFE INC.**

TIME-LIFE CUSTOM PUBLISHING
Vice President and Publisher: Terry Newell
Associate Publisher: Teresa Hartnett
Director of Editorial Development: Jennifer Pearce
Vice President of Sales and Marketing: Neil Levin
Director of Special Sales: Liz Ziehl
Director of New Product Development: Quentin McAndrew
Managing Editor: Donia Ann Steele
Production Manager: Carolyn M. Clark
Quality Assurance Manager: James King

Books produced by Time-Life Custom Publishing are available at
special bulk discount for promotional and premium use. Custom
adaptations can also be created to meet your specific marketing
goals. Call 1-800-323-5255.

Library of Congress Cataloging-in-Publication Data
Do-it-yourself health: 1,001 tips you can use to feel
better and stay well/by the editors of Time-Life Books.
p. cm.
Includes bibliographical references and index.
ISBN 0-7835-4939-3 (softcover)
1. Self-care, Health.
I. Time-Life Books.
RA776.95.D6   1997
362.1·'75 — dc21   97-10716 CIP

EDITORIAL STAFF

EDITOR
Robert Somerville

Deputy Editor
Tina S. McDowell

Design
Dana R. Magsumbol

Text Editor
Jim Watson

Associate Editors/Research and Writing
Stephanie Summers Henke
(principal)
Nancy Blodgett

Graphic Layout
Rebecca Mowrey

Copyeditor
Jayne Rohrich Wood

Picture Coordinators
Ruth Goldberg, Kim Grandcolas

Editorial Assistant
Patricia D. Whiteford

SPECIAL CONTRIBUTORS
Monika Thayer (design)
Patricia Daniels, Darcie C. Johnston,
Deborah Papier, Susan Perry,
James S. Thornton (text)
Lina B. Burton (index)

CONSULTANT
Jeffrey Migdow, MD

Jeffrey Migdow has been practicing holistic medicine for 17 years. In his medical practice, Dr.
Migdow counsels patients on lifestyle and recommends a wide variety of homeopathic, nutritional,
and other therapies. He is a medical consultant for the Health for Life Program and a director of
yoga-teacher training at the Kripalu Center for Yoga and Health in Lenox, Massachusetts. He
began his yoga training more than 20 years ago and has been teaching yoga for 10 years.

Introduction

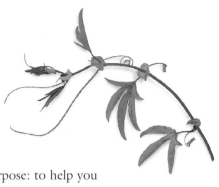

This book has a simple purpose: to help you take control of your own health. And the medicine it dispenses is knowledge. Unlike other health tips books, *Do-it-Yourself Health* offers you a complete package. You'll find many easy, practical things you can do at home, including a wide range of alternative therapies, from herbs to acupressure and yoga. But you'll also get valuable information on conventional care—when you need to see the doctor and what to expect when you're there. The operating principle in all cases is: what's best for your own and your family's health.

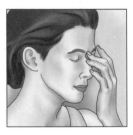

Organized by topics that range from general guidelines on good health to specific advice on a variety of health matters, *Do-it-Yourself Health* guarantees that you'll always be able to find the information you need in a flash. Having it at hand may very well be your first step toward better health.

Do-it-Yourself HEALTH

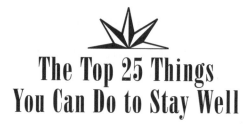

The Top 25 Things
You Can Do to Stay Well

SIMPLE

STRAIGHTFORWARD

STRATEGIES FOR

MAINTAINING A

HEALTHY BODY, MIND,

AND SPIRIT

The Top 25 Things You Can Do to Stay Well

TIP 1

TO LIVE HEALTHY, ADOPT HEALTHY HABITS

In a landmark 10-year study, Dr. Lester Breslow of U.C.L.A. found that men and women who practice seven common-sense health habits enjoyed longer lives and less disability than those who took their health for granted. What are these magic keys to health? Chances are you've already heard them—from your mom:

- Don't smoke.
- Keep your weight under control.
- Eat breakfast.
- Don't snack between meals.
- Be physically active.
- Don't have more than two alcoholic drinks per day.
- Sleep 7 to 8 hours a night.

TIP 2

E IS FOR EXCELLENT SUPPLEMENT

Though most nutritionists recommend a healthy diet as the main source of necessary vitamins and minerals, a daily multivitamin supplement can act as an insurance policy for occasional dietary gaps. One antioxidant in particular, vitamin E, has emerged as a great potential aid to the heart—most likely because it prevents the oxidation of low-density lipoprotein (LDL), or "bad" cholesterol, into a more dangerous form. Unlike most vitamins, however, it is almost impossible to obtain the recommended levels of vitamin E from diet alone. Many physicians now recommend a 400 IU supplement once a day.

TIP *3*

GET 25 PERCENT OF DAILY CALORIES FROM BREAKFAST

Make each meal you eat, including breakfast, account for at least one quarter of your daily calories. Some people divide breakfast-lunch-dinner "25-25-50." Others prefer to use a "30-40-30" split. Whatever your pattern, follow it consistently for about three weeks and your appetite will naturally "lock on" to the routine. Then you can forget about counting calories: Your appetite will guide you like an autopilot.

TIP *4*

WATER, WATER EVERYWHERE

Drinking plenty of water each day bestows multiple health benefits. Water helps curb appetite, serves as a natural laxative, lubricates joints, reduces wrinkling, prevents kidney stones and urinary tract problems, and can even ease a hangover.

TIP *5*

ALCOHOL: HEALTHY FOR SOME

Heavy drinking raises blood pressure, damages the liver, and increases the risk of multiple other health problems, from strokes and automobile accidents, to cancers of the colon and esophagus. For many people, however, researchers have found that alcohol in moderation can actually improve health by reducing stress and elevating blood levels of high-density lipoprotein (HDL), or "good" cholesterol. The key word here is moderation. For some people, two drinks a day is too many; for others, two (but no more) may be right. But if one drink affects your thinking process, alcohol's not a good idea for you.

TIP 6

KEEP YOUR VESSELS CLEAR

Make sure you know not only your overall cholesterol level but also your levels of LDL (the "bad" cholesterol that clogs vessels), HDL (the "good" cholesterol that helps clear out clogs), and the ratio of total cholesterol to HDL (less than 4 is ideal). If your lipid profile needs improvement, avoid saturated and "partially hydrogenated" fats, both of which cause LDL cholesterol levels to soar. Choose instead monounsaturated fats like olive or canola oil; these lower LDL without also depressing HDL. Eating onions and garlic can help raise HDL.

TIP 7

FEAST ON FLAVONOIDS

Antioxidant compounds called flavonoids, which are found in many fruits and vegetables, offer a host of health benefits. Flavonoids in grape skin, for instance, reduce blood cholesterol, and flavonoids in onions help prevent gum disease. Those found in cherries, blackberries, and blueberries may stave off macular degeneration, the leading cause of vision loss. Flavonoid supplements even seem to help kids with ear infections. Try a dose of 50 mg for every year of your child's age, up to 250 mg maximum. Even more promising: Researchers suspect that these biochemical wonders may reduce the risk for certain cancers, slow down the aging process, and boost immunity.

TIP 8

FIBER WITH AN EXTRA BOOST

Eating plenty of water-soluble fiber such as oat bran and psyllium seeds (found in many bulk-forming laxatives) can help protect you against heart disease. Soluble fiber works in your intestinal tract by binding to—and removing—building blocks for cholesterol. Insoluble fiber, such as the kind found in grains, whole wheat bread, beans, and many fruits and vegetables, is also important. Indeed, all fiber promotes regularity, speeds transit time through the digestive tract, and reduces the risk of colorectal cancer. The National Cancer Institute recommends consuming at least 25 grams of fiber each day.

TIP 9

AN ASPIRIN A DAY

If aspirin was discovered today, it would be hailed as a breakthrough miracle drug. Researchers have found that besides its ability to reduce pain and inflammation, a low daily dose can slash heart attack risk and possibly prevent polyps in the colon from turning cancerous. Aspirin does have side effects, however; most common are stomach irritation and possibly an increased risk of stroke. Check with your doctor before you opt for long-term use.

TIP 10

TO GET FIT, THINK F.I.T.

If you'd like to improve aerobic fitness, remember these three basic aspects of any exercise program:

Frequency: Exercise three or four times a week.

Intensity: Very light exertion won't cut it, but you don't need to exhaust yourself, either. Strive to reach a level that you perceive as somewhat hard.

Time: Spend at least a half hour on each workout.

TIP *11*

COPY CATS

Want to preserve a certain feline grace as you age? Use a cat for your role model. Slow, catlike body stretching before vigorous physical activity warms up muscles, helps prevent injuries, boosts muscle strength, enhances flexibility, and increases your range of motion. Try this yoga pose.

Cat

On your hands and knees, exhale as you arch your back, stretching your shoulder, neck, and back muscles. Inhale and bring your back to the horizontal.

TIP *12*

STRENGTH TRAINING

It's never too late to enjoy the considerable advantages that come from weight training. A study of 90-year-old men and women in a nursing home found they increased muscular strength by an average of 174 percent in eight weeks. Strength training not only builds stronger muscles, it increases bone density, boosts metabolic rate, and retards the aging process. For these and other benefits, the American College of Sports Medicine now recommends that all adults strength train at least twice a week. Just make sure a trainer shows you the proper techniques.

TIP *13*

AVOID "SMOKER'S FACE"

Want to avoid looking old before your time? Stop smoking now. Dermatologists can usually tell at a glance which of their patients are heavy smokers. The reason: Nicotine and other components in cigarette smoke constrict blood flow to the face, wreck the skin's natural elasticity, trigger premature wrinkles, and turn skin pale and sallow—a condition referred to as "smoker's face." If avoiding cancer, heart disease, and impotence isn't enough motivation to quit, try looking in the mirror.

TIP *14*

SAFETY FIRST

The quickest way to lose your health: a major accident. The Bureau of Safety Statistics and the National Transportation Safety Board recently reported the grim statistics: 46,000 Americans are killed each year in auto accidents; and 22,500 die from injuries sustained at home, another 12,000 from falls, and 5,000 from fires. For young men, accidents are the third leading cause of premature death and disability. One of the single best things you can do to guard your health is to adopt a "safety first" mindset. Conduct your own safety audit, then take the positive steps, from always wearing seatbelts to installing smoke detectors in your home, that can cut your risks.

TIP *15*

WEAR YOUR OWN SHADE

Skin cancer is the single most common form of cancer, and a deadly form of it—malignant melanoma—is growing at rates that astonish researchers. Damaging ultraviolet radiation is the chief culprit, but you can protect yourself without completely shunning the sun by making sure to protect all exposed skin with sunscreen. Choose a lotion that shields against both UVA and UVB rays and has an SPF (sun protection factor) rating of 15 or more.

TIP *16*

THE ABCD TEST

Check your skin once a month for melanoma. Moles that definitely warrant a doctor's immediate scrutiny have any or all of the following characteristics:

- Asymmetrical shape.
- Borders that aren't regular.
- Color variations.
- Diameter larger than a pencil eraser.

TIP *17*

CULTIVATE CLOSE RELATIONSHIPS

Sharing your concerns with loved ones, friends, or a support group of others with a common problem can make a tremendous difference in not only your psychological functioning but your immune response. Studies of women with breast cancer, for example, have found that joining a support group significantly enhances the odds of long-term survival.

TIP *18*

FRIENDS NEED NOT BE HUMAN

Researchers looking for ways to prolong survival in heart attack patients have found that the best medicine of all may walk on four legs. Patients who developed a close relationship with a dog, cat, or other pet animal recovered significantly faster and lived longer than those who lacked this bond. The likely explanation: By providing unconditional affection, pets reduce stress levels in their owners.

TIP *19*

PERIODIC CHECKUPS

It's a lot easier to treat a disease detected early than one caught late. For this reason, all adults should have regular checkups by their primary care physician. Along with a physical exam and family history, your healthcare provider will check blood pressure and cholesterol, take blood and urine samples for analysis, and may run other basic tests. Women over the age of 18, for instance, should get a yearly Pap smear. Men at 50 need an annual rectal exam, supplemented by a PSA blood test, to detect early signs of prostate cancer. Your doctor can explain these and any other tests you might need, and advise you on when you need to return for your next checkup.

TIP *20*

IMMUNIZATION IS NOT JUST FOR KIDS

Even if you received all your childhood inoculations, it's important to have tetanus and diphtheria booster shots every 10 years
throughout your lifetime. Moreover, two infections—pneumonia
and influenza—kill tens of thousands each year. If you're over 65
or suffer health problems that dampen your immune system, get
vaccinated against these potential killers. Alternatively, see a holistic practitioner, who will suggest other tactics for strengthening
your immune system.

TIP *21*

KNOW THE SIGNS OF DIABETES

Chronic thirstiness, frequent urination, tiredness, and sudden
weight loss can all be red flags for diabetes. See your doctor if you
experience two or more of these symptoms or if diabetes runs in
your family. Type II diabetes, the form that most often comes on
in adulthood, can sneak up on you. Indeed, up to half of all people with this disease don't know they have it.

TIP *22*

LAUGH YOURSELF HEALTHY

Laughter, it turns out, really is one of the best medicines.
Researchers have found an hour of chortles reduces stress hormones, fends off disease by activating T cells and other immu-
nological warriors, elevates brain awareness, and even increases
blood levels of natural painkilling opioids.

TIP *23*

MUSIC SOOTHES

A recent study found that 3 out of 4 women going through labor reported significantly less pain when music was being played. Other researchers have found that music can be a surprisingly potent cure for stress and anxiety—decreasing heart rate, blood pressure, and the levels of stress hormones in the blood.

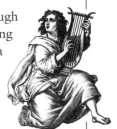

TIP *24*

THINK "WELL," FEEL BETTER

Researchers have found that the way you choose to view your own health can become a self-fulfilling prophecy. Optimists who adopt a positive outlook are sick much less often than pessimists who assume and expect the worst. One tip to try: When times get tough, focus on a past achievement. Then tell yourself you triumphed over adversity before—and you can definitely do it again.

TIP *25*

HEALTH FROM A HIGHER POWER

Scientific studies have long shown that faith and prayer can help boost overall health. Religious beliefs are an important source of inspiration for many people, but you don't necessarily need to adhere to a given faith to find solace. You can also benefit from a compassionate and forgiving outlook on life, a search for meaning and purpose beyond the circumstances of the moment, and the ability to surrender health problems to a higher power—and trust in the outcome.

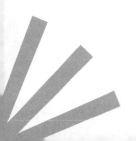

Dealing with Common Ailments

AN ALPHABETICAL

GUIDE TO TREATING

AND PREVENTING

COMMONPLACE

PROBLEMS—FROM ACNE

AND ATHLETE'S FOOT

TO WARTS AND

WHEEZING

———————

Dealing with Common Ailments

Acne

TIP 26

ZINC RELIEF

When acne flares up, nutritionists generally suggest zinc, which plays a part in how the body processes hormones. A 30- to 50-mg zinc supplement daily may help reduce inflammation and heal damaged skin.

Athlete's Foot

TIP 27

HOT SOCKS

Your coach and the school nurse were on the right track when they made you wear shower shoes in the locker room and around the pool. Other sensible steps for avoiding athlete's foot:

- Wear cotton socks, and shoes that breathe; shoes that keep water out also keep sweat in.
- Never share shoes, socks, or towels.
- If you get athlete's foot, wash your socks and towels in the hottest water possible—or boil them!

Bad Breath

TIP 28

FRESH FOODS, FRESH BREATH

A high-fiber diet with plenty of whole grains, fresh fruit, and raw leafy vegetables not only helps good digestion, but also reduces the chance of bad breath. Eating apples, oranges, and celery can help by cleaning the teeth, dispersing bacteria in the mouth, and stimulating saliva flow. Try chewing fresh parsley or peppermint leaves, a method used by ancient Romans to sweeten their breath.

Bad Breath

TIP 29

BRUSH YOUR TONGUE

For sweeter breath, clean your tongue as well as your teeth.
Brush the top of the tongue as far back as possible. A tongue
blade, a device used in the Middle East and India to scrape
the tongue, may be helpful. A soup spoon will work just as
well; gently draw the inverted bowl of the spoon over your
tongue to scrape off any residue. But be careful: Don't push
the brush, spoon, or scraper so far back that you start to gag.

Bee Stings

TIP 30

A MUD "BANDAGE"

If you are stung by a bee or a wasp, and the stinger remains in
the skin, scrape it away with a knife or a fingernail; if you use
tweezers, you may squeeze more venom into the skin. For bee
stings, a paste of baking soda will ease the itching. Wasp stings
are alkaline and can be neutralized by vinegar or lemon juice.
If you're far from home, apply mud; as it dries, it will draw
out some of the toxin.

HONEYBEE

WASP

Bee Stings

TIP 31

DON'T BE A FLOWER

Reduce your chances of being stung by avoiding brightly
colored, white, or pastel clothing. Don't use cosmetics
or perfume with floral scents. Food odors attract insects,
too, especially yellow jackets, so be alert when you are
cooking or eating outdoors.

YELLOW JACKET

TIP 32

NATURAL DEODORANTS

Tablets containing chlorophyll, a natural plant product, are sold as a deodorant that can be taken orally. Dusting the underarms and toes with baking soda, a good natural deodorant, also helps absorb odor. Crystallized mineral salts to control body odor are sold in health and cosmetic stores.

TIP 33

FIGHTING CANKER SORES

Canker sores, possibly caused by stress, generally go away by themselves. To relieve the discomfort, look for a medicine that contains glycerin, which protects the sore, and peroxide, which fights bacteria.

TIP 34

TEA BAGS TO THE RESCUE

Try applying a used black tea bag to your canker sore. The tea contains a natural astringent called tannin, which may ease the pain.

TIP 35

BE WARY OF REBOUND

When you're suffering from a miserable cold, it's tempting to dose yourself with one of the many over-the-counter "cold and flu" preparations, but think twice. These multisymptom drugs likely contain medications for symptoms you don't have, and therefore may result in needless overtreatment. Some drugs, such as decongestants, can cause a "rebound effect" if used for more than five days, making your congestion even worse than before.

Common Cold **TIP 36**

STEAM POWER

Herbal steam can reduce congestion, and if the vapor temperature is 110° F or higher, it will also kill cold germs on contact. Choose eucalyptus *(Eucalyptus globulus)*, wintergreen *(Gaultheria procumbens)*, or peppermint *(Mentha piperita)*. Place either fresh leaves or a few drops of the herb's oil in a bowl and pour in boiling water. Place a towel over your head, lean over the bowl to create a steam tent, and breathe the vapors.

PEPPERMINT

Common Cold **TIP 37**

JUMP-START YOUR IMMUNE SYSTEM

Taken at the first sign of cold symptoms, echinacea *(Echinacea* spp.) can reduce a cold's intensity and duration, often even preventing it from becoming a full-fledged infection. Echinacea apparently stimulates the immune response, enhancing resistance to all infection. This herb is available in capsules or as a tea.

>**Tea:** *Add 2 tsp echinacea root to 1 cup water; simmer for 15 minutes. Drink three cups daily.*

Common Cold **TIP 38**

HERBAL BREW

For a good "cold tea," combine equal parts of elder *(Sambucus nigra)*, peppermint *(Mentha piperita)*, and yarrow *(Achillea millefolium)* and steep 1 to 2 tsp of the mixture in 1 cup hot water. This blend can help the body handle fever and reduce achiness, congestion, and inflammation.

TIP *39*

GRANDMA WAS RIGHT

"Jewish penicillin," also known as chicken soup, has been heralded as a cold therapy since the 12th century. Recent scientific evidence supports the notion that chicken soup reduces cold symptoms, especially congestion. Something (yet to be determined) in the chicken soup keeps neutrophils from clumping together and causing inflammation.

TIP *40*

CHINESE OR MEXICAN?

If you're still hungry after that chicken soup, pick up some spicy Chinese or Mexican food. The hot stuff in the food can unclog even the stuffiest nose.

TIP *41*

TAKE YOUR VITAMINS

Good nutrition is essential for resisting and recovering from a cold. Eat a balanced diet. Take supplements as needed to ensure you are receiving the recommended dietary allowances for vitamin A, the vitamin B complex (vitamins B_1, B_2, B_5, B_6, folic acid), and vitamin C, as well as the minerals zinc and copper. If your diet is deficient in zinc, your body is low in neutrophils, and you're an easy mark for all types of infections, including colds. And because zinc apparently kills viruses on contact, sucking zinc lozenges can also help shorten the duration of colds or viral sore throats.

Common Cold **TIP 42**

COLD MYTHS AND FACTS

Contrary to myth, you cannot catch a cold by being cold, or by getting wet, or by sleeping near an open window. Colds are caused by viruses, and these viruses are most commonly spread by direct contact. Don't share towels, silverware, or beverages with someone who has a cold. Cold viruses often survive for hours in the open, on doorknobs, money, and other surfaces, so wash your hands frequently.

Corns and Calluses **TIP 43**

AN OVERNIGHT CURE

Hydrocortisone creams may help remove cracked calluses. Apply the cream and cover the area overnight with a plastic bag or a sock. In the morning, rub off as much of the callus as you can with a coarse towel or brush. Using a pumice to rub the dead skin from a callus after showering, then applying urea-based cream, can also be effective. Do not try this with corns; rubbing will just make them more tender and painful.

Cough **TIP 44**

DROWN A COUGH

Since coughing is a protective response by the body, doctors usually do not recommend suppressing it with cough medicine. The best thing to do for a cough is to drink plenty of liquids, four to six big glasses a day. A large intake of fluids will loosen the mucus and make coughing it up easier. Warm liquids, or just plain water, are best for the purpose. Try to avoid caffeinated or alcoholic beverages, which are diuretics that cause you to lose more liquid than you take in.

Cough **TIP 45**

PRESSURE AID

If coughing spasms become too bothersome, try acupressure: Pressing Lung 5 may help ease your cough.

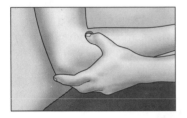

Lung 5
Bend your right elbow and make a fist. Place your left thumb on the outside crease (thumb side) of the elbow alongside the taut tendon and press firmly. Repeat on the other arm.

Earaches **TIP 46**

WHEN WAX IS TO BLAME

When excess earwax blocks the eardrum, it can result in earaches, ringing in the ears, and partial hearing loss. Try the following remedy: For three days, place a few drops of warm baby oil or mineral oil in the ear twice daily to soften wax. Then use a bulb syringe to flush out the wax with warm water. Note that you may feel some temporary dizziness.

Flu **TIP 47**

BOOST YOUR BODY'S RESPONSE

For the achy misery of influenza, try an herbal approach to stimulating your immune system. Take ½ tsp each of tincture of goldenseal *(Hydrastis canadensis)* and echinacea *(Echinacea* spp.) two times a day.

Gas Pains

TIP *48*

WATCH WHAT YOU EAT

Crampy gas pains are often caused by diet. When bothered by gas, try making changes in what you eat. Increase your fiber intake slowly and try avoiding beans, peas, and fermented foods such as cheese, soy sauce, and alcohol. Drink fewer carbonated drinks. Avoid mixing proteins and carbohydrates at the same meal. For people who are lactose intolerant, replacing cow's milk with soy milk may help.

Gas Pains

TIP *49*

SOME CLAY EACH DAY

For persistent gas, dissolve a teaspoon or two of superfine white, green, or yellow French clay (available at health food stores) in water and drink at least once daily (but not with meals). The clay absorbs impurities and intestinal gas; it also absorbs medications you may be taking, so don't take it within two hours of when you take your medicine.

Hangover

TIP *50*

THE MORNING AFTER

Instead of "the hair of the dog" (yet more alcohol), try the following diet to help you recover from a hangover. Nutritionists recommend fruit juices diluted with water or seltzer, and consumed at two times the volume of the amount of alcohol you have drunk; crackers and honey to ease nausea; and bouillon to restore salt and potassium levels.

TIP 51

HERBAL DO'S AND DON'TS

To relieve the symptoms of hay fever and other allergies, take two capsules of nettle *(Urtica dioica)* every 15 minutes during an attack, then four times a day as a maintenance dose. Many herbalists have also found success with ephedra *(Ephedra sinica)*, but you should not treat yourself and should take it only under the supervision of a qualified practitioner; ephedra can cause dangerous side effects, including heart palpitations and high blood pressure, and has even caused fatalities when taken improperly.

TIP 52

POURING PAIN AWAY

Your imagination can sometimes be the best medicine for a headache. Try this technique, which relies on your mind's own power to overcome pain. It helps to have a partner talk you through the exercise, but with practice you may be able to do it yourself.

Close your eyes and imagine that your headache is a liquid that fills a certain size of container—the more painful the headache, the bigger the container. Now imagine pouring your headache pain into a slightly smaller container, without letting any of the liquid overflow. Keep pouring the liquid into smaller and smaller containers; bit by bit, you should feel the pain reducing.

TIP 53

FOOD TABOOS FOR MIGRAINES

Among the foods sometimes associated with migraine headaches are chocolate, aged cheeses, citrus fruits, processed meats containing sodium nitrates or the food additive MSG, and red wine. Keeping a food diary can help you identify foods to eliminate.

Headaches

TIP 54

MIGRAINE RELIEF

If your migraines are mild and occur less often than three times per month, your doctor may suggest drugs such as ergotamine or an isometheptene-containing combination. The drug suma-triptan, available in tablet or injectable form, is designed to treat migraines and brings dramatic relief.

Headaches

TIP 55

DEFUSING TENSION HEADACHES

To stop a tension headache, try the following exercises while breathing deeply and thinking calmly. While seated, inhale and gently tip your head back until you're looking at the ceiling. (Be careful not to tip your head back too far; this can compress the cervical spine.) Exhale and bring your head forward until your chin rests on your chest; repeat twice. You can also try pressing Gall Bladder 20 for relief.

Gall Bladder 20
Place the tips of your middle fingers in the hollows at the base of your skull, about two inches apart on either side of the spine. Press firmly.

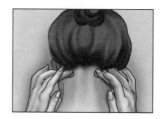

Headaches

TIP 56

FOR FREQUENT MIGRAINES

Doctors prescribe a wide range of medications for migraines. If you have three or more severe, prolonged migraines per month, your doctor may suggest using preventive medications on a continual basis. These include propranolol, a beta-adrenergic blocker that works by reducing constriction in blood vessels; a calcium channel blocker such as verapamil; or low-dose antidepressants.

TIP 57

FOODS TO AVOID

Despite its name, heartburn has nothing to do with the heart. If the lower esophageal sphincter (LES), the valve between the esophagus and stomach, opens too often or too far, stomach acid can seep into the esophagus and cause a burning sensation. If you have frequent heartburn, avoid foods that relax the LES, including tomatoes, citrus fruits, garlic, onions, chocolate, coffee, alcohol, and peppermint.

TIP 58

SOOTHING TEAS

According to herbalists, ginger *(Zingiber officinale)* tea can diminish heartburn quickly, and chamomile *(Matricaria recutita)* tea's calming effects are especially helpful for stress-related heartburn.

TIP 59

SIT IN A SITZ

It's an old remedy, and it still works like a charm: For the pain and itching of hemorrhoids, take a sitz bath. Sit in about three inches of warm (but not hot) water for 15 minutes, several times a day, especially after a bowel movement. (If you are pregnant, discuss any treatment with your doctor before proceeding.)

TIP 60

REDIRECT THE BLOOD FLOW

To encourage blood flow away from hemorrhoids, thereby reducing pain, inflammation, and bleeding, try lying on a slant board with your head downward for 15 minutes each day.

TIP 61

A TEA BREAK FOR HICCUPS

To stop the hiccups, herbalists recommend warm chamomile
(Matricaria recutita) tea, which is said to act as an antispasmodic
agent. Another remedy that might bring relief is a tea
that combines peppermint *(Mentha piperita)*, boneset *(Eupatorium perfoliatum)*, cayenne *(Capsicum
annuum* var. *annuum)*, and lemon.

> ***Tea:*** *Mix ½ tsp of tinctures of peppermint and
> boneset with a few drops of cayenne and the juice of
> a quarter lemon in 1 cup hot water.*

TIP 62

SEVEN HICCUP-BUSTERS

The goal of any of these cures is either to override or to disrupt
the nerve impulses that cause the hiccups. Here are some sugges-
tions that may help you interrupt the hiccup cycle:

- Place a tsp of sugar under the tongue and let it dissolve slowly; or swallow the sugar dry.
- Bend forward from the waist and drink water from
  the opposite side of a glass.
- Tickle the roof of your mouth with a cotton swab at
  the point where the hard and soft palates meet.
- Hold your breath and swallow at the same time you
  feel the urge to hiccup. You may need to repeat this
  two or three times until your hiccups cease.
- Place a brown paper bag over your mouth and
  breathe forcefully and rapidly into it at least 10
  times. Be sure the seal around your mouth is tight so
  no outside air gets in.
- Suck on a lemon wedge soaked in angostura bitters
  or sprinkled with cayenne, or swallow 1 tsp vinegar.
- If your child has the hiccups, tickle him gently while
  instructing him to hold his breath and not to laugh.

Hives **TIP 63**

HIVES BEGONE

One of the best remedies for hives is a soothing bath.

> **Bath:** *Add 5 or 6 tbsp oatmeal, 3 tbsp cornstarch or sodium bi-carbonate, or a strong infusion of chickweed to your bathwater.*

Hypoglycemia **TIP 64**

BOOST YOUR BLOOD SUGAR

For mild cases of hypoglycemia—low blood sugar—eat small, frequent high-protein meals. Supplements of chromium may help regulate blood sugar levels, whether they're low or high. Chromium can be found in brewer's yeast, whole-grain breads and cereals, molasses, cheese, and lean meats.

Indigestion **TIP 65**

PARK THAT GUM

If you frequently chew gum—and also find yourself suffering from indigestion—quit the gum habit for a while to see if your symptoms dissipate. It's common to swallow air when chewing gum, which can cause indigestion.

Ingrown Nails **TIP 66**

LEMONY TOES

If ingrown nails are paining you, try this natural remedy: Tie a fresh lemon slice—a softening agent—around the affected toe and leave it on overnight. When the nail is pliable enough to ease out of the flesh, trim it, and then put a thin strand of sterile cotton under the corner to lift it away from the skin until it grows out. Change the cotton daily.

Insect Bites

TIP 67

STOP BUGS FROM BUGGING YOU

Essential oil of eucalyptus *(Eucalyptus globulus)* is a natural insect repellent.

Solution: Add 5 drops of essential oil of eucalyptus to a cup of almond or olive oil, and dab on your skin.

Insect Bites

TIP 68

TRY AN ASPIRIN

For minor insect and spider bites, some doctors suggest rubbing the bite with an aspirin that has been crushed and moistened with a few drops of water.

Jock Itch

TIP 69

BOXERS, NOT BRIEFS

If you have been prone to jock itch in the past and normally wear briefs, consider switching to boxer shorts, which can help keep the groin area drier by allowing better air circulation.

Lice

TIP 70

AN HERBAL RINSE

To treat the all-too-common affliction of head lice, aromatherapists recommend washing the hair and rinsing slowly with a pint of warm water containing 6 drops each of essential oils of rosemary *(Rosmarinus officinalis)* and red thyme *(Thymus vulgaris)*. Dry the hair naturally (not with a blow dryer), then comb with a special fine-toothed comb designed to remove louse eggs that cling to hairs. For prevention, soak your comb in water with 10 drops of essential oil of red thyme, and comb hair thoroughly.

TIP 71

PUTTING MOTION SICKNESS TO REST

Ginger *(Zingiber officinale)* is a favorite motion sickness remedy of naturopathic physicians. It causes none of the side effects of antinausea drugs and can be drunk as a tea, eaten candied, or taken in capsule form (two capsules every four hours the day before and as needed during travel); take on an empty stomach.

TIP 72

PREVENTING CRAMPS

If you get frequent nighttime cramps, nutritionists recommend taking vitamin E supplements (300 IU daily). You may also find relief by increasing your intake of calcium. Good sources include milk, cheese, yogurt, dark green leafy vegetables, and canned fish.

TIP 73

UNTYING A KNOTTED MUSCLE

To relieve a typical cramp, you need to make the muscle stop contracting—by physically either stretching it or massaging it, or both. You can stretch a calf muscle simply by standing on your toes and then slowly lowering your heels. For a greater stretch, put your hands or forearms against a wall and, keeping your feet flat on the floor, slide backward until you are leaning against the wall from several feet away. For even more stretch, keep edging your feet backward.

Poison Ivy — TIP *74*

ANTIDOTE PLANTS

The leaves of jewelweed *(Impatiens)* which often grows near poison ivy, may neutralize the plant's burning oil, urushiol. Try wiping the leaves over the skin right after contact. You might also try a few drops of juice squeezed from the leaves of the common plantain *(Plantago major)*.

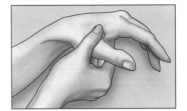

POISON IVY

Sneezing — TIP *75*

APPLY THE PRESS

To help stop fits of sneezing, press Large Intestine 4, located in the web between the thumb and index finger.

Large Intestine 4
Use the thumb and index finger of your right hand to squeeze the webbing between the thumb and index finger of your left hand for one minute. Switch hands and repeat. (Do not apply pressure to this point if you are pregnant.)

Snoring — TIP *76*

STOP THE RACKET

While heavy snorers will snore in any position, moderates tend to snore only when sleeping on their backs. One way to avoid this is to sew a pocket onto the back of your nightclothes and insert a tennis ball, which will make it uncomfortable for you to lie on your back and prompt you to turn on your side during sleep.

Sore Throat　　　　　　　TIP *77*

SLIPPERY ELM FOR SORE THROATS

To ease the discomfort of a sore throat, try this traditional Native American treatment.

> **Tea:** *Put 2 tsp powdered slippery elm (Ulmus fulva) bark in 1 cup water. Bring to a boil and simmer for 10 to 15 minutes.*

Sore Throat　　　　　　　TIP *78*

HOMEMADE GARGLES

To wash away mucus and irritants and bring relief from the pain of a sore throat, try any of the following gargles:

Salt water: Mix ½ tsp salt in 8 oz warm water.

Sage: Put 1 to 2 tsp dried leaves in 1 cup boiling water; steep for 10 minutes, then strain and cool until lukewarm.

Horseradish: Mix 1 tbsp pure horseradish, 1 tsp honey, and 1 tsp ground cloves in 8 oz warm water.

Sunburn　　　　　　　TIP *79*

AFTER SUNBURN

The best source of relief is to apply aloe vera gel to burned areas. A cool bath laced with several tablespoonfuls of baking soda or cider vinegar can relieve the pain, itching, and inflammation of a moderate sunburn.

Aloe

Sunburn

TIP 80

COOL CUCUMBERS

For particularly sore spots of sunburn, try applying sliced cucumber, apple, or potato to the afflicted area. They soothe the burn and may help ease inflammation.

Warts

TIP 81

A FOLK CURE THAT WORKS

There are countless folk cures for warts. One that may have some validity is rubbing the wart with a slice of raw potato or the inner side of a banana skin; both contain chemicals that may dissolve the wart.

Wheezing

TIP 82

WHEEZING AND YOGA

Make sure you see a conventional doctor to determine the cause of your wheezing. However, some alternative therapies can help ease the discomfort. Try, for instance, the yoga position known as the cobra.

Cobra
Place both forearms on the floor, elbows directly under your shoulders. Slowly straighten your arms and arch your back until your abdomen is off the ground. Relax and slowly uncurl, lowering your torso back to the floor.

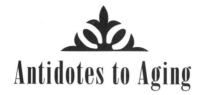

Antidotes to Aging

PREVENTIVE

TECHNIQUES

TO HELP YOU

STAY YOUNG—

AND TO KEEP YOU

WELL AS YOU AGE

Antidotes to Aging

TIP 83

REMEMBER YOUR GINKGO

Help keep your memory young with a daily dose of ginkgo biloba
extract (GBE). Studies have shown that gingko improves blood flow to the brain, so this herb may also
help prevent a stroke—and the memory loss, vertigo,
and depression that may follow one. The recommended average dose is 40 mg, taken three times a
day, or 15 drops of ginkgo tincture, taken twice a day.

GINKGO

TIP 84

A SUPPLE REMINDER

Keep your joints loose and limber—and help ease the stiffness
that comes with age-related arthritis—by performing gentle yoga
stretches on a regular basis.

TIP 85

RUB OUT VARICOSE VEINS

If varicose veins are a worry, massage oil of rosemary into the
legs to stimulate circulation. Oils of cypress and chamomile may
soothe swelling and inflammation and help relieve pain.

TIP 86

SHADES TODAY, CLEAR TOMORROW

To keep cataracts from clouding your vision when you're older,
wear sunglasses that filter out harmful UVB rays. Use them even
on a bright but cloudy day.

TIP 87

RELIEF FOR SORE EYES

Use hydrotherapy to stimulate circulation in the eyes and reduce the stress and eyestrain caused by overworked eyes and middle-age diseases like glaucoma: Alternate hot and cold compresses for three minutes each, three times a day.

TIP 88

WALK AWAY
FROM CONSTIPATION

Before you reach for a laxative to relieve constipation, try walking it off. Regular exercise is an excellent way to correct chronic constipation and carries none of the possible side effects of laxatives, which can damage the lining and injure the nerves of the colon.

TIP 89

GET A MOVE ON

Regular exercise, a healthful diet, and at least eight glasses of water a day will help you avoid constipation—and hemorrhoids—as you grow older.

TIP 90

GO WITH GRAIN

To help prevent diverticulitis—a disease of the intestines and colon that becomes more common with age—increase your intake of fiber and water, and engage in regular exercise.

TIP 91

WATCH NOW FOR DIABETES

To minimize your chances of contracting adult onset (Type II) diabetes, maintain a proper weight for your height, exercise, and eat a nutritionally balanced diet.

TIP 92

QUIT AND CALM DOWN

Keep your skin youthful—and lessen your chances of developing emphysema as you age—by kicking the smoking habit. To aid relaxation during nicotine withdrawal, try meditation, guided imagery, biofeedback, and soothing herbs such as chamomile *(Matricaria recutita)* and valerian *(Valeriana officinalis)*.

VALERIAN

TIP 93

GET THE GOUT OUT

If you suffer from gout, which afflicts mostly middle-aged men, drink an infusion of 2 tsp celery seed *(Apium graveolens)* or gravelroot *(Eupatorium purpureum)* in a cup of water, three times a day, in order to rid the body of excess uric acid. (**Caution:** Do not drink herbal teas if your doctor has prescribed colchicine.)

TIP 94

MASSAGE FOR GREAT GUMS

To keep gums young, protect them against infections, and speed healing, massage them regularly with vitamin E oil or poultices of myrrh *(Commiphora molmol)* or goldenseal *(Hydrastis canadensis)*.

MYRRH

TIP *95*

FLOWER UP YOUR SMILE

To reduce the bacteria that may cause gum disease, massage your gums with calendula *(Calendula officinalis)* tincture, made from marigold flowers.

TIP *96*

TOE TRICKS FOR HEALTHIER FEET

Prevent the foot problems that often arise with age by strengthening your feet now. One clever exercise: Learn to pick up objects with your toes.

TIP *97*

HAIR TOMORROW?

To stimulate your scalp and help promote new hair growth, use a tonic made from traditional Chinese herbs such as polygonum *(Polygonum multiflorum)*, lycium fruit *(Lycium barbarum)*, Chinese foxglove root *(Rehmannia glutinosa)*, Chinese yam *(Dioscorea opposita)*, or cornus *(Cornus officinalis)*. You can also try horsetail *(Equisetum arvense)* herbal drops to strengthen roots and promote growth; take 15 drops twice a day.

HORSETAIL

TIP *98*

DON'T BE A FLAKE

Help prevent the dry, flaky skin that comes with age—and strengthen fragile hair—by massaging your scalp with a few drops of vitamin E oil or flaxseed oil.

TIP 99

HEAR YE, HEAR YE

Some kinds of hearing loss may be lessened by reducing the
amount of salt in your diet. Excess salt causes a buildup of fluids in
the ear, which can put pressure on delicate hearing mechanisms.

TIP 100

IS THAT THE PHONE?

To treat hearing loss—particularly if it is accompanied by a ringing or roaring in the ears—try vitamin A supplements, 5,000 to
10,000 IU a day.

TIP 101

BUILDING STRONGER ARTERIES

To tone and strengthen your arterial walls—and help avoid
aneurysms and strokes—see a homeopathic professional about
a preventive remedy called *Baryta carbonica*.

TIP 102

EATING FOR SELF-DEFENSE

A healthy immune system is your best defense against many of
the ills that strike with age. Good dietary practices, such as getting the recommended daily dosages of vitamins A, B complex,
C, and E, and the minerals zinc and selenium, will keep your
immune system strong. Vitamins A, C, and E, along with additional fruits and vegetables in the diet, may fight the aging
effects of free radicals—unstable molecules in the body that can
harm cells—which some studies have linked to nerve damage
and vision problems.

TIP *103*

WARM UP TO ROMANCE

Aging needn't mean giving up your sex life. Take turns slowly and lightly touching and caressing each other to renew sexual interest.

TIP *104*

PUT THE SQUEEZE ON INCONTINENCE

Growing older may bring incontinence, especially for women. Spending minutes a day contracting muscles that control urination can strengthen them and alleviate, or greatly control, the problem.

TIP *105*

LOVE YOUR LIVER

For a healthy liver, limit alcohol consumption, avoid uncooked shellfish, and ask an herbalist about milk thistle *(Silybum marianum)*, a plant believed to promote healthy liver function.

MILK THISTLE

TIP *106*

VITAMIN E PROTECTION

Menopause and hormone replacement therapy may increase a woman's risk for breast cancer and other breast problems. Experts recommend taking at least 400 IU daily of vitamin E as protection.

TIP *107*

BABY YOUR NAILS

Maintain healthy, supple nails with herbs and minerals. Try taking horsetail *(Equisetum arvense)* (15 drops twice a day) and 30 to 40 mg of zinc regularly.

TIP *108*

A DANDY WAY TO WEED OUT SWEETS

To avoid gaining weight in middle age, add dandelion *(Tarax-acum officinale)* leaves to your salad, or brew them in a tea; this may help boost your metabolism and reduce a craving for sweets.

TIP *109*

HERBS THAT HELP PREVENT BONE LOSS

To help slow the progression of bone loss that occurs during the aging process and that sometimes leads to the weakened bone condition known as osteoporosis, try these herbs in tea or tincture form: horsetail *(Equisetum arvense)*, alfalfa *(Medicago sativa)*, licorice *(Glycyrrhiza glabra)*, marsh mallow *(Althaea officinalis)*, or sourdock *(Rumex crispus)*. Several Chinese herbs, most notably dong quai *(Angelica sinensis)* and Asian ginseng *(Panax ginseng)*, are also recommended for preventing bone loss. HORSETAIL Consult a practitioner experienced in Chinese herbal medicine for appropriate dosages.

TIP *110*

EXERCISE FOR STRONG BONES

You need to get moving to reduce bone loss and prevent osteoporosis. But not all movement is the same. To keep bones strong, you must do weight-bearing exercises—those that put stress on bones, such as running, walking, tennis, ballet, stair climbing, aerobics, and weightlifting. And you must do the exercises at least three times a week for 30 to 45 minutes. Swimming and bicycle riding, although good cardiovascular exercises, do not appear to prevent osteoporosis because they do not put enough stress on bones.

TIP 111

EAT MORE CALCIUM-RICH FOODS

To retain calcium in your bones and thus keep them from thinning and weakening as you age, you may need to increase the amount of calcium in your diet. If you are an adult male, you should be getting 800 mg of calcium in your diet daily. If you are a woman, you should be getting 1,000 mg of calcium daily—or 1,500 mg if you are postmenopausal and not taking estrogen supplements. Healthful, calcium-rich foods include nonfat milk, low-fat yogurt, broccoli, cauliflower, salmon, tofu, sesame seeds, almonds, and leafy green vegetables. At the same time, avoid foods that can interfere with your body's absorption of calcium, such as red meats, soft drinks, and excessive amounts of alcohol and caffeine.

TIP 112

ZINC ON THE HALF SHELL

As men grow older, they become more prone to prostate problems. To maintain a healthy prostate, eat oysters—a rich source of zinc, which is thought to promote prostate health and reduce inflammation.

TIP 113

HERBS FOR THE PROSTATE

To keep the prostate gland healthy and reduce mild inflammation, try herbal therapies—such as an extract of the berries of the saw palmetto tree *(Serenoa repens),* found in the American Southeast, or Asian ginseng *(Panax ginseng),* or flower pollen.

SAW PALMETTO

TIP 114

SKIN CARE BEGINS WITH 'B'

Slow the hands of time and keep your skin healthy and glowing with regular supplements of vitamin B complex.

TIP 115

HELP FOR THIN SKIN

To enhance collagen production and repair connective tissue— components of the skin that break down over time—ask a professional about supplementing your intake of vitamins C, B_6, and E, as well as zinc.

TIP 116

STRIKE BACK AT STROKES

Reduce your risk of stroke—most common in people over the age of 60—by eating a low-fat diet rich in such stroke-deterring nutrients as potassium, magnesium, vitamin E, and the essential fatty acids contained in fish oils.

TIP 117

NUTRITION FOR YOUR BLADDER

The risks of bladder cancer increase as we age. Take preventive steps by adding vitamin B_6, beta carotene, and selenium to your diet. Fresh fruits and vegetables are the best sources.

TIP *118*

A VEIN EFFORT

Since veins weaken with age, start now to strengthen them. Certain yoga positions, including the Plow, Corpse, and Half Shoulder Stand, increase circulation and drain extra blood from the legs, keeping veins supple.

Plow
While on your back, inhale and raise both legs, using your hands to support your hips. Exhale as you try to touch the floor behind you with your toes. Stretch out your arms on the floor, then place your hands back on your hips and slowly lower your legs.

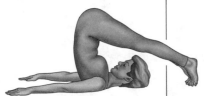

TIP *119*

FIGHT PLAQUE WITH GARLIC

Eating large amounts of garlic *(Allium sativum)* may help reduce the plaque deposits in blood vessels that lead to hardening of the arteries.

TIP *120*

EYEBRIGHT FOR A SHARPER IMAGE

To slow age-related vision loss, strengthen your eye tissue by taking 2 or 3 capsules of eyebright *(Euphrasia officinalis)* every day.

TIP *121*

DISSOLVE WARTS WITH PINEAPPLE

Rid your skin of the warts that often appear as skin ages by using this folk-medicine remedy: Soak a cotton ball in fresh pineapple juice, which contains a dissolving enzyme, and rub it on the wart.

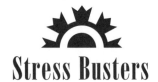

Stress Busters

REMEDIES AND
ROUTINES TO DESTRESS
YOUR DAY AND YOUR
LIFE—INCLUDING TIPS
FOR KEEPING
WORK WORRIES
AT A DISTANCE

Stress Busters

TIP 122

THE RELAXATION RESPONSE

Try the relaxation response for stress relief: Sit quietly, relax your body, breathe slowly and deeply, and say "peace" or "I'm calm" each time you exhale. Don't try to chase thoughts out of your head; in fact, don't try to do anything. Practice for five minutes at a time, gradually building up to one or two 20-minute sessions per day. When performed regularly, the relaxation response slows breathing, calms brain-wave patterns, and lowers blood pressure.

TIP 123

RELAX WHEN YOU'RE SICK

Don't stop eliciting the relaxation response just because you're suffering an illness. Not only will relaxation help you handle the stress of being sick, but it can also give a boost to your immune system and speed your recovery.

TIP 124

STRESS RELIEF
ENDS WITH A FROWN

Relieve stress by contracting then relaxing your muscles in sequence. Begin by contracting the muscles in your toes as hard as you can, for 10 seconds, then relax them for 10 seconds. Work your way up your body, through all your major muscles—feet, legs, torso, fingers, arms, neck, and face.

TIP *125*

TRY BIOFEEDBACK

Learning biofeedback from a skilled professional equipped with the right monitoring devices can let you control a host of so-called autonomic physiological functions, from body temperature to gastrointestinal function to the electrical activity in your brain. Once you learn how, you can practice at home without equipment. Ask your family doctor for a referral.

TIP *126*

COPY A CORPSE

The Corpse is an excellent yoga position for relaxing.

Corpse
Lie on your back, with your feet about 18 inches apart and turned out slightly. Place your hands about 6 inches from your hips, palms up. Close your eyes and breathe deeply.

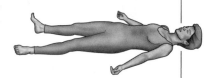

TIP *127*

FIGHT OR FLIGHT SIMULATOR

Use high-intensity exercise, from punching a body bag to going for a long run, to do what stress has geared your body to do: fight or flee. Stress triggers the release of pulse-quickening hormones; vigorous aerobic exercise can reduce the level of these hormones.

TIP *128*

UNLEARN HURRY AND WORRY

Avoid the learned behaviors of hurry and worry, which can upset your sleep and meal schedules and cause your stress level to spiral upward. Remind yourself that you'll accomplish more in the long run if you pace yourself and accept your own limitations.

TIP *129*

COMPLEMENTARY HOBBY

The best way to unwind is to choose an enjoyable after-hours activity that offers different challenges from your work. For instance, if you have a desk job, try losing yourself in a physical hobby like gardening. If your job tends to isolate you from other people, pick a social hobby like playing cards.

TIP *130*

STRESS AUDIT

Divide all the stresses in your life into two categories: those you can do something about, and those that are out of your control. Work on handling the first type—and ignore or avoid the others whenever possible.

TIP *131*

TAKE VACATIONS

Make periodic time away from work a priority: Don't just pay lip service to a need to get away "sometime." If leaving the office behind is difficult for you, keep reminding yourself that a little time off to recharge your batteries will make you more productive in the long run.

TIP *132*

MIND TRIPS

When you're feeling overwhelmed in a stressful environment, use guided imagery to take a brief mental vacation to a favorite setting, such as a secluded beach. Close your eyes and focus on all five senses to vividly bring your sanctuary to life. You might also try supplementing your psychic escape with some soothing music.

TIP *133*

STRESS IS CUMULATIVE

Pay attention to—and work to resolve—the little aggravations in your life. It's not just the big stresses like divorce or a major illness that can threaten your sense of well-being. Seemingly trivial stressors can add up fast.

TIP *134*

A REASONABLE SCHEDULE

Rational time management is a key to reducing stress. Write down everything you feel must get done, then prioritize the items from most important to least. You'll make faster headway, and feel a lot less stressed, if you work down from the top priorities and strive never to overbook yourself.

TIP *135*

WISDOM FROM THE BARD

Try to gain a positive perspective on a stress in your life. The same event that paralyzes one person can inspire another. As Shakespeare wrote: "There is nothing either good or bad, but thinking makes it so."

TIP *136*

A FRIENDLY PRESENCE

If you're nervous about a medical test or a public-speaking engagement, take a friend along. Having a friend by your side can take the edge off a stressful event. Researchers have also found that the physical proximity of a friend lowers your blood pressure and heart rate.

TIP *137*

TEAM UP
WITH YOUR COMPETITORS

If you're a cutthroat Type A competitor, force yourself to do something nice for a rival. You may just find that a "joining them" mindset is much less stressful than a "beating them" attitude—and less stress will make you ultimately more effective.

TIP *138*

WHEN STRESS
IS A FAMILY AFFAIR

Learn to resolve conflicts with your spouse peacefully, for your own sakes and for your children's. Researchers have found that parental fights increase behavioral and emotional problems in children, which only ratchets up everyone's stress levels further.

TIP *139*

A BUFFER ZONE
BETWEEN WORK AND HOME

A half hour's exercise after work, a short nap, even quiet reading can all create a defensive wall to keep your work stresses from spilling over into your home life.

TIP 140

TIDY UP YOUR STRESS

A neat home and office can eliminate that out-of-control feeling. Psychologists have found that for many men and women, the actual process of tidying up can reduce stress and anxiety.

TIP 141

DRESS DOWN
TO STRESS DOWN

Change into comfortable clothing as soon as you can after work. A change in fashion is a great way to separate yourself psychologically from the stresses of the work environment.

TIP 142

SHARE HOME WORK

Discuss the manifold jobs of your household, from cooking and cleaning, to child care and home maintenance. Devise a division of domestic labor that feels fair to every family member—and post a schedule on your refrigerator.

TIP 143

BE REAL ABOUT CHORES

Be willing to compromise on your standards for housekeeping. Your kitchen floor doesn't have to be clean enough to eat off. Slightly lowering standards can remove lots of stress.

TIP *144*

KEEP THE INSTRUCTIONS HANDY

Always store the instructions and warranty information for household products in a single place in your home. That way, the information will be at your fingertips when you need it—and you won't ever find yourself searching in a panic when something goes wrong.

TIP *145*

MASSAGE AWAY STRESS PAINS

If stress causes you physical symptoms like headache, neckache, or backache, try a professional massage followed by self-massage of your temples, face, neck, and shoulders.

TIP *146*

REAL HELP WITH HYPNOSIS

Try self-hypnosis to relieve the stress-related condition known as irritable bowel syndrome. A recent study found that hypnosis can significantly relax painful colonic contractions.

TIP *147*

SHORT-TERM RELIEF

Ask your doctor about the short-term use of anti-anxiety medications when an acute situational stress, such as a death in the family, is making it hard for you to function. Prescription drugs like alprazolam are safe and effective when taken over a period of no more than a few weeks. A natural anti-anxiety medication is Bach flower essence called Rescue Remedy. Herbalists recommend taking a few drops every couple of hours.

TIP *148*

A BREATH OF PEACE

Try putting 2 to 3 drops of essential oil of lavender *(Lavandula officinalis)* on a handkerchief and inhaling from this when you're feeling stressed. Some people also find it relaxing to place 5 to 6 drops in a warm bath.

TIP *149*

STRESS-BUSTING TEAS

For soothing relief for stress-frazzled nerves, try a warm cup of herbal tea. Teas made from chamomile *(Matricaria recutita)*, passionflower *(Passiflora incarnata)*, valerian *(Valeriana officinalis)*, or ginseng *(Panax quinquefolius)* can all be relaxing. Find the one that works best for you.

PASSIONFLOWER

TIP *150*

BEAT NERVES WITH B'S

If stress is leaving you jumpy, try a daily supplement of vitamin B_6, which can help nervousness, insomnia, and tremors. Vitamin B_{12}, which can calm generalized anxiety and reduce heart palpitations, may also help.

TIP *151*

PRESSURE POINTS

If you find that acupuncture helps relieve stress for you, learn which acupuncture points work best to relax your body. Use a whirlpool jet or a friend's fingertips to massage these points daily.

TIP *152*

DO THE TWIST

A great yoga posture for relaxing is the Knee Down Twist.

Knee Down Twist

Lie on your back with your arms out. Inhale and place your right foot on your left knee. Exhale, then turn your head to the right and bring your right knee toward the floor to your left (right). Release slowly, then repeat on the other side.

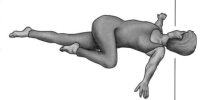

TIP *153*

RIDE THE BUS

If you're prone to teeth-grinding at every highway bottleneck, try a different route: Take public transportation instead. If you have to, you can work on your way to work. Better still: Read a book for pleasure and arrive relaxed. Even the walk to and from the bus stop is a good way to stress-relieve your commuting.

TIP *154*

PACKED AND READY

Frequent business travelers can minimize the stress of last-minute trips by keeping a fully packed suitcase ready to pick up and go at a moment's notice.

TIP *155*

IN FLIGHT EXERCISE

If fear of flying has got you down, let off nervous energy by doing discreet stretching and isometric exercises with your seatbelt on and your seatback upright. For example, place your elbows on the armrests and push down as hard as you can, hold for 10 seconds, relax, then repeat.

TIP *156*

A PIECE OF HOME

Lower the stress of business travel by carrying along a reassuring reminder of home. Family pictures in the wallet are a common such reminder, but don't feel you have to limit yourself. A surprising number of business travelers report packing their suitcases with such domestic comforts as a night light, a security blanket, or even a teddy bear.

TIP *157*

COLOR YOURSELF UNSTRESSED

Surround yourself with cool colors to soothe and relax your system. Bright, vibrant hues are great for energizing you, but it's best to avoid these when trying to relax.

TIP *158*

INSPIRING ART

Decorate your work space with personally meaningful photographs or paintings that inspire and relax you. From natural landscapes to abstract art, visual images exert a strong influence on mood.

TIP *159*

FIGHT STRESS WITH STRESS

Put yourself to the test by enrolling in a program that presents real physical challenges. Successful participation in high-stress, white-knuckle sports like rock climbing and white-water rafting can show you your inner strength in the face of adversity. This, in turn, can help you take more down-to-earth stresses in stride.

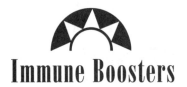

Immune Boosters

HELPING YOUR OWN

DEFENSE FORCES

STAY IN PEAK

FIGHTING FORM WITH

NUTRITION, HERBS,

MIND/BODY MEDICINE,

AND MORE

———————

Immune Boosters

TIP *160*

VITAMIN C

Enhance your immune system by eating foods rich in vitamin C —such as citrus fruits, bell peppers, and leafy greens—or by taking vitamin C supplements, from 500 mg to 2,000 mg each day. Megadoses (more than 1 gram) of vitamin C may lessen the duration and the severity of cold symptoms, as well as help prevent infections and cancer.

TIP *161*

CONEFLOWER TEA

Drink echinacea (*Echinacea* spp.) tea, three times a day, to enhance your resistance to bacterial and viral infections. The dried root of this popular perennial, known as the coneflower, is available in dried form in bulk, and in capsules, tea, and tincture.

Tea: Add 2 tsp echinacea root to 1 cup water; simmer for 15 minutes.

ECHINACEA

TIP *162*

PUT ZINC IN YOUR DIET

To boost your immune system's resistance to all types of infections, eat plenty of zinc-rich foods, such as lean meats, seafood, eggs, and soybeans, or take a daily multinutrient supplement that includes zinc chelate, zinc picolinate, or zinc aspartate. This essential mineral is also available as a tablet or throat lozenge.

TIP *163*

THE HERB, NOT THE CANDY

Pump up the power of your immune system in its fight against invading microbes with marsh mallow *(Althaea officinalis)*. The roots of this plant, which is unrelated to the campfire candy named marshmallow, contain a spongy substance that is believed to support immune cells in their fight against invading microbes.

MARSH MALLOW

TIP *164*

PUNGENT POWER

Add garlic *(Allium sativum)*, raw or cooked, to your diet to boost your immune system and to help fight infections. Or take up to 4 capsules of powdered garlic or garlic oil each day. Applied externally, garlic is believed to help kill fungal infections, such as ringworm and athlete's foot.

GARLIC

TIP *165*

SOUTH AMERICAN CURE

Try pau d'arco *(Tabebuia impetiginosa)* to help your immune system fight fungal, bacterial, viral, and parasitic infections. The pau d'arco tree, also called the trumpet tree, is native to Central and South America and to the West Indies; it can reach a height of 125 feet. Take 15 drops of pau d'arco tincture, twice a day, or drink 2 cups of pau d'arco tea daily.

ᴛɪᴘ *166*

VIRAL RESISTANCE

To fight viral infections and enhance the functioning of immune cells, herbalists recommend taking astragalus *(Astragalus membranaceus)*. This herb contains substances known as polysaccharides, which are believed to stimulate the immune system and generally strengthen the body, speeding metabolism, promoting tissue regeneration, and increasing energy. Astragalus is available as prepared tea, fluid extract, capsules, and dried root.

Tea: *Boil 1 oz astragalus root in 1 cup of water for 15 to 20 minutes.*

ᴛɪᴘ *167*

FLU IMMUNITY

Protect yourself from the flu during flu season by gargling with a mixture of 1 drop each of the essential oil of tea tree (*Melaleuca* spp.) and lemon in a glass of warm water; stir well before each mouthful. Or take ½ tsp each of goldenseal *(Hydrastis canadensis)* and echinacea (*Echinacea* spp.) tinctures twice a day.

GOLDENSEAL

ᴛɪᴘ *168*

VACCINATION

To lower your chances of catching the flu, consider getting vaccinated. Though the vaccine is not without risks and it only protects against certain, selected flu viruses, it is especially recommended for the elderly or anyone with a chronic medical condition that would make the bug particularly hazardous.

TIP *169*

ANTIBACTERIAL TEA

Drink myrrh *(Commiphora molmol)* tea, three times a day, for this herb's infection-fighting ability. Myrrh battles infections by stimulating the production of immune cells, and by a direct antibacterial action.

Tea: Steep 1 to 2 tsp of powdered myrrh per cup of boiling water for 10 to 15 minutes.

MYRRH

TIP *170*

NATURAL ANTISEPTIC

Experts recommend the use of calendula *(Calendula officinalis)*, commonly known as marigold, to help fight infections and boost the immune system. A natural antiseptic and anti-inflammatory agent, it is one of the best herbs for treating wounds, skin abrasions, burns, bug bites, and infections. Calendula is available in lotions, ointments, oils, tinctures, and fresh or dried leaves and florets.

CALENDULA

TIP *171*

HAPPINESS AND HEALTH

Feel good about yourself. It's true: Stress depresses immunity, and feeling good strengthens it. One study discovered that the impact of positive experiences such as expressions of love or feelings of accomplishment continues for two days, whereas the effects of negative events such as criticism or arguments last only one day. This suggests that the affirming consequences of happiness are more powerful and longer lasting than the negative effects of sadness—by 2 to 1.

TIP 172

AEROBIC EXERCISE

To help your immune system, try walking for 45 minutes, five times a week. Vigorous aerobic exercise can reduce the level of pulse-quickening hormones released during stress and stimulate a sense of well-being. Even a walk around the block can help to reduce anxiety or let off steam.

TIP 173

IMAGINE YOUR WAY TO HEALTH

If your immune system has become depressed from tension buildup, try this visualization exercise: Close your eyes and cover them with your hands. Concentrate on filling your visual field completely with blackness, then invite yourself to see a color you associate with stress; next, substitute that color in your mind's eye with one you perceive as soothing—replacing red with blue, for example. A variation on this technique might be to picture a tense scene, such as a traffic jam, and replace the image with a calmer one, such as a lake or meadow.

TIP 174

BATHE YOUR STRESS AWAY

Use hydrotherapy to alleviate your stress, which in turn will help your immune system: Hormones released by the body during stress depress the immune system. Soak for 10 to 20 minutes in a tub of very warm water, using half a cup of Epsom salts and your favorite bath oil. Or add 1 drop each of the essential oil of lavender, jasmine, or German chamomile to the bathwater.

LAVENDER

TIP *175*

YOGA BENEFITS

Strengthen your immune system and increase your vitality with yoga. These relaxation exercises slow your breathing rate, decrease your oxygen consumption, calm your brain-wave rhythms, and lower your blood pressure. Two positions that are especially helpful to the immune system are the Child and the Bridge.

Child

Sit on your heels, knees together. With your arms at your sides, palms up, bend from the hips and extend your upper body over your knees, bringing your forehead toward the floor. Then slowly sit up.

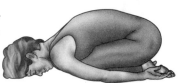

Bridge

Lie on your back, knees bent, palms on the floor. Tense your buttocks and slowly raise your pelvis. Clasp your hands, arching as you press your shoulders to the floor. Hold this position, then unclasp your hands and slowly lower your pelvis to the floor.

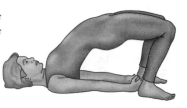

TIP *176*

TIME-PROVEN WISDOM

Relax with a cup of hot chamomile tea *(Matricaria recutita)*, and energize your immune system in the process: Chamomile has been used for centuries for its relaxing qualities and immunity-boosting benefits.

> ***Tea:*** *Pour 8 oz of boiling water over 2 tsp chamomile flowers and steep for 10 minutes. Drink 1 cup three or four times daily.*

CHAMOMILE

TIP *177*

ACUPRESSURE BOOST

Applying gentle pressure to the acupressure point called Gall Bladder 20 may help strengthen your immune system while relieving fatigue and depression.

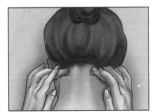

Gall Bladder 20
Place the tips of your middle fingers in the hollows at the base of your skull, about two inches apart on either side of the spine. Press firmly.

TIP *178*

A MUSHROOM A DAY

To stimulate the immune system and help maintain good health, eat one shiitake *(Lentinus edodes)* mushroom a day; you can incorporate shiitakes into a wide variety of recipes. Chinese medicine practitioners recommend eating two to four ounces of shiitake mushrooms two or three times a week for general health benefits. These mushrooms contain oligosaccharides, known to be extremely potent immune stimulators.

TIP *179*

FREE RADICAL PROTECTION

Daily doses of Asian ginseng *(Panax ginseng)* or dried ginkgo *(Ginkgo biloba)* may improve immune system functioning by protecting against the damaging effects of free radicals—unstable molecules that can harm cells.

GINKGO

TIP *180*

QUIT FOR YOUR IMMUNITY

One good thing you can do for your immune system is to eliminate chronic, nagging challenges to it. This is but one more reason to stop the cigarette habit. Smoking assaults mucous membranes and the lungs, increasing your susceptibilty to all sorts of respiratory infections—which can make your immune system work harder than it needs to.

TIP *181*

COMMON SENSE

To promote good health, examine your habits and make changes if necessary: Avoid overeating and overindulging in alcohol, caffeine, and tobacco. Exercise regularly, and eat a balanced diet.

TIP *182*

SLEEP IS KEY

Set up a regular sleeping schedule and get plenty of rest—without sleeping pills. If you need help falling asleep, try an herbal tea made with valerian *(Valeriana officinalis)*, passionflower *(Passiflora incarnata)*, hops *(Humulus lupulus)*, or skullcap *(Scutellaria lateriflora)*.

VALERIAN

TIP *183*

HEALTHY BACTERIA

To make sure that your digestive tract contains healthy bacteria, eat a cup of plain yogurt daily or pick up *Lactobacillus acidophilus* supplements from your health food store. Sometimes these bacteria are killed when you take certain antibiotics, or they become overwhelmed by other intestinal flora.

TIP *184*

SUPPLEMENTAL AID

Keep your immune system strong with good dietary practices, such as getting the recommended daily dosages of vitamins A, B complex, C, and E, and zinc, selenium, and other trace minerals. Take a daily antioxidant multivitamin containing the U.S. recommended daily allowance of these nutrients.

TIP *185*

HELPING IMMUNITY HELP YOU

Try to avoid taking antibiotics, unless your doctor recommends them: The immune system grows stronger with every battle won, so helping it fight with remedies less powerful than antibiotics— such as analgesics, vitamins, and herbs—will allow the immune system to do its job.

TIP *186*

CHINESE REMEDY

Dried slices of the Chinese remedy known as polyporus, from the mushroom *Polyporus umbellatus*, can be made into a tea and drunk for a tonic effect on the immune system.

TIP *187*

A FRIEND IN NEED

In times of illness or trauma, social support is crucial. People with close personal relationships are the most likely to recover from serious illness or injury. The ability to form relationships with people—or pets, for that matter—can be a key to good health.

TIP *188*

PROTECT YOURSELF

As much as possible, avoid radiation exposure, harmful chemicals, and prolonged use of immunosuppressive drugs such as corticosteroids, all of which can impair immunity.

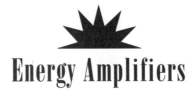

Energy Amplifiers

Ways to restore
youthful vigor,
get the most
from your
sleeping hours,
and keep daily
fatigue at bay

———————

Energy Amplifiers

TIP 189

STRENGTHEN INTERNAL ENERGY WITH T'AI CHI

Take a class in this ancient Chinese practice at your local YMCA, health club, or Taoist center. A martial art form that combines slow-motion movements and meditation, t'ai chi helps many practitioners feel calm and invigorated.

TIP 190

PROTEIN FOR BREAKFAST

Add three ounces of protein to your breakfast menu, especially on days when you know you'll need to concentrate deeply for extended periods. Protein boosts a brain chemical that's necessary for sustained mental alertness. But be aware that protein in the morning can make some people feel exhausted; if this happens to you, try other energy-amplifying strategies.

TIP 191

A BREATH OF ENERGY

Try this quick and rejuvenating breathing exercise: Exhale completely through your mouth, inhale through your nose to the count of four, hold your breath for a count of seven, exhale through your mouth for a count of eight. Repeat three times whenever you need an energizing pick-me-up.

TIP *192*

CURING THYROID LOWS

Fatigue can come from a low level of thyroid hormones. Increase your production of thyroid hormones with supplements of vitamin C, vitamin E, riboflavin (vitamin B_2), zinc, niacin (vitamin B_3), pyridoxine (vitamin B_6), and tyrosine.

TIP *193*

WAKE UP YOUR BRAIN

Take 15 drops of ginkgo *(Ginkgo biloba)* tincture in the morning. This herb increases blood flow to the brain, which can help you wake up and get energized.

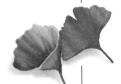

GINKGO

TIP *194*

CULTIVATING ENERGY

Learn and practice qigong ("chee-goong") daily to boost energy levels and overall health. This ancient Chinese discipline, which translates as "energy cultivation," uses the multiple repetition of deceptively simple exercises to balance the body's energies and promote wellness.

TIP *195*

RAG DOLL RELAXATION

To regain lost energy, try a yoga exercise called the Rag Doll.

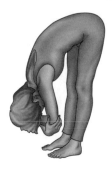

Rag Doll

Standing with arms at your sides, exhale and bend forward from the hips, letting the top of your head drop toward the floor. Cup your elbows in your palms and breathe deeply. Slowly stand up, bringing your head up last.

TIP *196*

ANTIDOTES FOR CHRONIC FATIGUE

For relief from the symptoms of chronic fatigue, take the nutritional supplement coenzyme Q10, vitamin B_{12}, the herb gotu kola *(Centella asiatica)*, and a combination of malic acid and the mineral magnesium.

TIP *197*

DRAINED BY DRINKING?

If you want to be energetic tomorrow, don't drink too much alcohol today. Drinking interferes with the digestive absorption of folic acid, which is necessary for the production of red blood cells that are critical to your energy level.

TIP *198*

FATIGUE IN THE MEDICINE CABINET

If you're feeling tired all the time, check your prescription and over-the-counter medications. Common culprits known to induce fatigue include antihistamines, cough suppressants, and blood pressure pills. Your doctor can usually switch you to an effective alternative without this side effect.

TIP *199*

TIME THE LIGHT

Reset your body's internal clock by exposing yourself to plenty of natural light during the daytime—and turning your lamps to low in the evenings, especially before bedtime. Light stops the release of the hormone melatonin, which helps you sleep.

TIP *200*

RELIEF FROM JET LAG

If international business travel has sent your body clock haywire, minimize the energy drain by making sure to keep your body well hydrated. Drink plenty of water—and avoid alcohol. Bach flower Rescue Remedy, taken every hour on the plane, can help reset your body's internal clock.

TIP *201*

DOWN AND UP

Go to bed only when you're sleepy, but get up each morning at the same time no matter what your bedtime. Eventually, your body will lock on to the wake-sleep schedule it needs for optimal daytime energy.

TIP *202*

SUGAR AND SLEEP

A light starchy snack before bed will stabilize blood sugars while you sleep. Choose a baked potato, slice of bread, an apple, or other complex carbohydrate, but avoid sweets and fruit juices because these can gyrate blood sugar levels and disrupt sleep.

TIP *203*

NO TO A CAFFEINE NIGHTCAP

Avoid coffee, tea, and caffeinated soft drinks for several hours before bedtime. Beware of hidden caffeine as well: Chocolate contains caffeine, and many over-the-counter medications—including commonly used pain relievers—have caffeine as an ingredient.

TIP *204*

TIMING EXERCISE

Find your own best time of day for workouts. For many people, exercise is both relaxing and energizing, which can be a problem if you work out too close to bedtime. For most, exercising in the morning or afternoon guarantees daytime energy and tiredness at the right time—in the evening.

TIP 205

AVOID OVERSTIMULATION
AT BEDTIME

The same advice that applies to toddlers applies to adults as well: Don't get all revved up right before bed. Avoid discussing, for instance, hot topics like money. As the Bible says, "The pursuit of money chaseth away sleep." Try instead 15 minutes of quiet conversation, light reading, or soft music.

TIP 206

A CHAMOMILE NIGHTCAP

A hot cup of bedtime tea made from chamomile *(Matricaria recutita)* helps many people find their way to sleep. Other strategies include a warm bath or deep breathing.

CHAMOMILE

TIP 207

CURE THE SNORE

If you are frequently tired during the daytime, your problem could be heavy snoring at night. People who suffer from a severe form of snoring called sleep apnea actually stop breathing repeatedly during the night, which turns a restful night's sleep into a battle for breath.

TIP *208*

A NEW
ANTI-INSOMNIA DRUG

If you suffer from insomnia, ask your doctor about a medication called zolpidem, which was introduced in 1993. Unlike older insomnia-fighting drugs, zolpidem has few side effects and doesn't induce "rebound" insomnia when discontinued. It is now the most commonly prescribed medication for the short-term management (7 to 10 days) of insomnia. It may be your answer to this energy-sapping problem.

TIP *209*

DIETARY SOPORIFIC

Try a turkey sandwich and a glass of warm milk as a bedtime snack. These foods are rich in the amino acid tryptophan, which plays a role in inducing sleep.

TIP *210*

MIMIC THE MOON

If you suffer from chronic fatigue, try the yoga exercise called the Half Moon.

Half Moon

Inhale and clasp your hands over your head. Exhale and stretch to the left, pushing out your right hip. Breathe deeply, keeping your shoulders and hips in the same plane. Inhale and return to the center. Repeat on the right side.

TIP *211*

CAFFEINE SUBSTITUTE

If caffeine makes you jittery, try inhaling peppermint oil instead, which provides an energy boost without coffee's buzz. If you get sleepy while driving, try a peppermint air freshener to keep you alert behind the wheel.

TIP *212*

RUN OFF THE BLUES

Run, swim, or participate in other vigorous aerobic exercise to restore energy sapped by depression. Regular exercise is a significant aid to recovering from—and preventing—depression.

TIP *213*

CLIMB THE MOUNTAIN

You can gain energy from a yoga position called the Mountain.

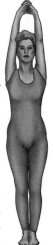

Mountain

Stand with your feet together. Inhale and raise your arms straight out from your sides, then join them over your head. To release, exhale and slowly lower your arms.

TIP 214

RULE OUT DISEASES

If you are constantly tired, see your doctor about possible physical causes for your fatigue, such as hypothyroidism, vitamin or iron deficiency, anemia, heart problems, and hidden cancer.

TIP 215

HEMORRHOIDAL FATIGUE

Treat severe hemorrhoids to restore energy. Hemorrhoids, stomach ulcers, and gastrointestinal tumors can all lead to chronic blood loss, resulting in anemia. Many other conditions, from dietary deficiencies to genetic defects, can also cause anemia. See your doctor for diagnosis and treatment.

TIP 216

THYROID HORMONE REPLACEMENT

You can treat the lethargy, reduced heart rate, insomnia, and other symptoms caused by an underactive thyroid by bolstering your body's low levels of thyroid hormone with a synthetic replacement such as the prescription drug levothyroxine. Ask your doctor if this drug is appropriate for your condition.

TIP *217*

SEAWEED RELIEF

If your energy problems are caused by an underactive thyroid, a tea made from the seaweed bladder wrack *(Fucus vesiculosus)* can help improve thyroid function.

Tea: Pour a cup of boiling water on 2 tsp of bladder wrack and steep for 10 minutes before drinking. Drink three times a day.

TIP *218*

FOODS TO AVOID

Enhance your body's ability to produce thyroid hormone by avoiding broccoli, cabbage, peaches, rutabagas, soybeans, spinach, peanuts, and radishes. All of these foods hinder the body's production of the hormone.

TIP *219*

THE PROBLEMS OF OVERTRAINING

Don't exercise to extremes. Workouts should leave you feeling invigorated, not exhausted. Too much of a good thing can lead to red blood cell "sports anemias," which can cause chronic tiredness, headaches, and increased susceptibility to infections.

TIP 220

LEAN ENERGY

If you're overweight and feeling sluggish, lose some pounds, counter stress with relaxation exercises like yoga, and get into the habit of working out regularly. The more energy you expend—without overdoing—the more energy you'll have.

TIP 221

NAPS CAN SAP

Avoid napping during the daytime to help ensure a good night's sleep and plenty of energy the following day. But if naps work for you, go right ahead. The important thing to remember is that the total amount of sleep you get in a 24-hour period is more important than when those hours come.

TIP 222

A FORMULA
FOR TIREDNESS

If you're suffering from ongoing fatigue, try a commercial mix of Chinese herbs called the Astralagus Ten Formula to help bring energy back. Consult an herbalist specializing in Chinese medicine for the proper dosages.

TIP *223*

PRESSURE
THE GALLBLADDER

If depression or chronic fatigue is sapping your energy, try applying gentle acupressure to Gall Bladder points 20 and 21.

Gall Bladder 20
Place the tips of your middle fingers in the hollows at the base of your skull, about two inches apart on either side of the spine. Press firmly.

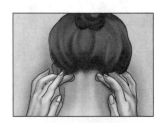

Gall Bladder 21
Apply pressure with your right middle finger to the highest point on your left shoulder muscle, one or two inches out from the base of the neck. Repeat on the other side. (Use light pressure if you are pregnant.)

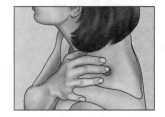

TIP *224*

GOTU KOLA

The herb gotu kola *(Centella asiatica)* naturally stimulates your adrenal glands, which can boost your energy levels. Herbalists recommend taking 15 drops of glycerated gotu kola tincture two times a day.

GOTU KOLA

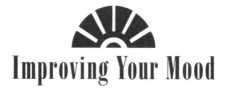

Improving Your Mood

EVERDAY STRATEGIES

FOR FIGHTING

THE BLUES,

OVERCOMING

ANXIETY,

AND NURTURING A

POSITIVE OUTLOOK

Improving Your Mood

TIP 225

WEAR MANY HATS

Take on many roles in your life. Spouse, parent, employee, coach, friend, mentor: Studies show that men and women who take on multiple roles are happier than those who focus their energies more narrowly.

TIP 226

SELF-AFFIRMATION

Compliment yourself from time to time. You can find favorite affirmations in poetry or prayers, or you can make up your own. Examples: "I feel good, I feel strong." Or, "I am a loving spouse and parent." Don't dismiss it as silly until you've tried it.

TIP 227

THE GOLDEN RULE OF COPING

Help your mate cope the way that works best for her or him, not for you. Many women prefer to talk out their problems, while many men prefer to distract themselves, at least initially.

TIP 228

REDUCING MOOD CONTAGION

Don't automatically blame yourself when a loved one is upset. Recognizing the real source of stress—a bad day at work, for example—can go a long way to preventing needless arguments that could send your own mood plummeting.

TIP 229

PRACTICE PARADOX

Experiment by going against your natural grain. If you find yourself overworked because of a need to control, try delegating a task. If you're always rushing, try getting in the longest waiting line at the bank.

TIP 230

STAY WELL
IN BODY AND MIND

If you want to be happy, take care of your physical as well as your mental health. As philosopher John Locke put it, "He that has these two has little more to wish for; and he that wants either of them will be little the better for anything else."

TIP 231

FIND THE FLOW

Find those pursuits at home and at work where you are most likely to experience flow—a sense of being caught up in the joy and excitement of the activity. Once you find the flow, go with it.

TIP 232

ROAD RUNNER IN THE A.M.

If you watch TV with your morning coffee, take a tip from your kids: Watch cartoons instead of the morning news shows. A jolt of a.m. levity will brighten your mood at work.

TIP *233*

JOKE TAPE

Buy audio tapes of stand-up comedians, and play one anytime you get caught in a traffic jam. Laughing creates a healthful state of "eustress" that is the opposite of "distress." Not only does it make you feel better, it may boost immunity and longevity.

TIP *234*

CONTAGIOUS JOVIALITY

Surround yourself with cheerful friends and avoid melancholy individuals. As Euripides put it, "Where there are two, one cannot be wretched and the other not."

TIP *235*

RECIPE FOR LAUGHTER

Now that you're in the working world, "school" can actually be your playtime. Take a fun course with a friend and find out how easily the laughter comes when, for instance, the two of you attempt to decorate your first cake.

TIP *236*

KEEP A JOKE JOURNAL

Jot down any good jokes you hear in a little notebook and share them with friends who have a similar sense of humor.

TIP *237*

PET ANTICS

Get a pet. Pets not only provide their owners with un-conditional positive regard, they're also funny. Ask any pet owner for some favorite stories, and prepare to hear an earful.

TIP *238*

RUNNER'S HIGH

Use endurance exercises to give your mood a great natural boost. Sustained aerobic exercise such as running or swimming can trigger the release of endorphins, the body's natural pain-killers. These not only relieve anxiety and depression, but they can also elevate an okay mood into the realm of feeling great.

TIP *239*

INOCULATE YOURSELF
WITH EXERCISE

Use regular, moderate exercise to erect a fire wall between you
and bad moods. For best results, work out aerobically at least
three times a week for 30 minutes or more.

TIP *240*

ALLEGRO OR PIANISSIMO

Use music to lead your mood where you want it to go. The
Moonlight Sonata, for instance, is great for relaxing. Try
the 1812 Overture for stress-free energy. Find the
tunes that work best for you, then make your own
"greatest hits" tape.

TIP *241*

WATERING YOUR MOOD

Take a bath or shower to adjust your mood from excitement
to relaxation—or vice versa. Cold water will definitely get you
going; warm water will let you relax before sleep.

TIP 242

THE 10 COUNT

Before lashing out in anger or self-defensiveness, take a deep
breath and slowly count to 10. It's an old trick but it really
works. A deliberate pause can be an instant tranquilizer.

TIP 243

MANY OPTIONS

Find one or two mind/body relaxation methods that work best
for you, then practice once or twice each day. A wide variety of
techniques have been proven to restore equanimity, from tran-
scendental meditation and yoga, to Oriental exercise techniques
like t'ai chi and qigong.

Corpse
*Lie on your back, with your feet about 18 inches
apart and turned out slightly. Place your hands
about 6 inches from your hips, palms up. Close
your eyes and breathe deeply.*

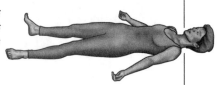

TIP 244

TARGET THE SYMPTOMS

Match relaxation techniques to your symptoms. If stressful situations make you physically jumpy, try exercise, yoga, or t'ai chi to
relax your body. If your symptoms are more mental, try meditation to quiet the mind and induce the relaxation response.

TIP 245

CALMING
ACUPRESSURE POINTS

If you want to induce a sense of peace in your body and your mind, try squeezing firmly for one minute on two acupressure points: Heart 7 and Pericardium 6.

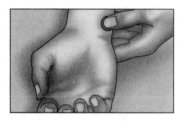

Heart 7
This point is located on the crease along the inside of the wrist, directly in line with the little finger. Squeeze firmly, using the thumb and index finger of your other hand.

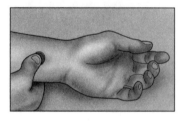

Pericardium 6
To find this point, measure two finger widths above the center of the wrist crease on the inside of your arm. With your thumb, press between the two bones of the forearm. Repeat on the other arm.

TIP 246

YOGA BREATHING

It is nearly impossible to be anxious when breathing deeply and slowly. Try the following exercise: Lie on your back, place one of your hands on your abdomen, then breathe in slowly and deeply through your nose. Your hand should be pushed up and out by your diaphragm as you inhale. Continue inhaling as deeply as possible, then reverse the process—exhaling slowly and completely. Repeat several times.

TIP 247

ESSENTIALS ONLY

Trim your schedule to the bare essentials, and whenever possible avoid putting yourself into nerve-racking situations. If, for example, tight deadlines throw you for a loop, make sure to plan ahead, start early, and avoid procrastinating.

TIP 248

AVOID THE RUT

Periodically change your daily routine to break monotony and provide a fresh perspective. This could be as simple as altering the route that you drive to work.

TIP 249

ATTITUDE ADJUSTMENT

Realize that success and happiness are not the same thing. Success is getting what you want; happiness is wanting what you get.

TIP 250

JOYFUL JOURNEY

Focus on the trip, not the destination. Most people get more fulfillment and satisfaction from striving to reach a goal than from actually reaching it. With this in mind, take time to regularly remind yourself to enjoy the ride.

TIP 251

NEITHER EASY
NOR IMPOSSIBLE GOALS

Set challenging but achievable goals—and periodically adjust these as circumstances change. Expecting little of yourself can make life seem dull and pointless, while striving for the impossible will leave you frustrated and feeling like a failure.

TIP 252

BATTERY RECHARGE

Learn how long you can work steadily before you need some time off. For many people, taking a long weekend every six weeks or so goes a long way to keeping burnout at bay.

TIP 253

THE PURSUIT OF HAPPINESS

Don't strive for personal happiness but rather work to make someone else happy. You'll find your own joy comes naturally along the way.

TIP 254

JOYFUL PROVERB

Embrace the wisdom of an ancient Chinese proverb: Happiness is having someone to love, something to do, and something to hope for.

TIP 255

RESET YOUR SET POINT

Put yourself in a position to enjoy many positive experiences. Each person's general degree of happiness, like his or her body weight, tends to hover around a "set point" that's influenced by heredity. Researchers have found, however, that you can adjust your set point by seeking out enjoyable and fulfilling activities.

TIP*256*

LOOK HAPPY, FEEL HAPPY

When you're feeling blah, try feigning the facial expressions of happiness. Method actors have used this technique for decades because it really works.

TIP*257*

A TIP FROM BEN FRANKLIN

Don't ignore the little triumphs in your life. As Benjamin Franklin put it, "Happiness is produced not so much by great pieces of good fortune that seldom happen, as by the little advantages that occur every day."

TIP*258*

DEFUSE HOSTILITY

If anger often sours your mood, ask yourself three questions whenever you feel hostility surging: Is it important? Am I justified? Can I do anything about it? If you answer yes to all three, go ahead and get mad. Otherwise, let it go.

TIP 259

THE POWER
OF DISTRACTION

When a problem in your life is bringing you grief, try gaining perspective by taking a break from your ruminations. Distractions such as a movie, a good book, or a game of basketball can give your mind something new to focus on. Later, when you return to your problem, chances are you'll see it in a much better light.

TIP 260

MAKING THE WORST OF IT

Minimize your worries by comically maximizing them. Example: Imagine a group of movie producers discussing whether or not to do a horror film about your upcoming dental appointment—and deciding against it because it would be just too grim for viewers to endure.

TIP 261

FLOODING WORRIES

If something is worrying you, vividly describe the problem on a cassette tape. Spare yourself no horrific detail. Make the problem as sickeningly gruesome as you can. Then listen to this tape several times a day until it starts to get boring and loses its power.

TIP*262*

WORRY WART REMOVER

If your ability to feel happy is hindered by chronic worry, try setting aside a "worry" period each day. For 15 minutes, concentrate on nothing but your worries; you may be surprised how hard it is to fill up the entire time.

TIP*263*

WRITE DOWN WORRIES

Jot your worries down—every one of them. Carry a pad of paper and pen, and any time you find yourself worrying, force yourself to write down the exact thoughts running through your mind. Eventually, you'll get sick of doing this—and you'll find it's easier to not worry than to keep up with the worry journal.

TIP*264*

SET YOUR FEARS TO MUSIC

A great way to defuse a fear is to sing it. For example, try singing the following lines to the tune of Beethoven's Fifth: "I'm out of cash; I'm going broke." Singing worries makes it hard to take them quite so seriously.

BEETHOVEN

ᴛɪᴘ*265*

BACH FLOWER REMEDIES

For a quick rescue from an anxious situation, place 1 to 10 drops of agrimony, aspen, and cherry plum into a beverage and drink as needed. Pioneered at the turn of the century by Edward Bach, these flower essences can be purchased at most health food stores.

ᴛɪᴘ*266*

HERBAL TRANQUILLITY

Restore your equanimity by drinking herbal teas. Chamomile *(Matricaria recutita),* lemon balm *(Melissa offici-nalis),* and linden *(Tilia* spp.) flowers are all mild but effective tranquilizers. If you need something stronger, try skullcap *(Scutellaria lateriflora),* valerian *(Valeriana officiualis),* hops *(Humulus lupulus),* and passionflower *(Passiflora incarnata).* All are available—with directions—at health food stores.

CHAMOMILE

ᴛɪᴘ*267*

MAGNESIUM MAGIC

Take magnesium supplements of no more than 300 mg three times a day for relief from anxiety, especially when this is accompanied by muscle cramps. Just don't take too much, which can lead to diarrhea.

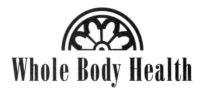

Whole Body Health

HEAD-TO-TOE

GUIDANCE FOR

THE HEALTH

OF YOUR BODY'S

MANY SYSTEMS—FROM

JOINTS, BONES, AND

MUSCLES TO YOUR

HEALTHY HEART

———————

Eyes, Ears, Nose, and Throat

TIP *268*

SOOTHING TIRED, ITCHY EYES

An eyewash made from the herb eyebright (*Euphrasia offici-nalis*) can help soothe strained or irritated eyes. It can also ease the itching and inflammation caused by conjunctivitis, commonly known as pinkeye.

Eyewash: Steep 1 tsp of the dried herb in 1 pt boiling water; then cool and strain. Using an eyecup, wash the irritated eye several times a day.

EYEBRIGHT

TIP *269*

PREVENTING PINKEYE

Bacterial conjunctivitis—or pinkeye—is highly contagious. The following preventive measures will help keep the condition from spreading to your other eye or to other people.

- Wash your hands often and well.
- Keep your hands away from the infected eye.
- Don't share washcloths, towels, pillowcases, or handkerchiefs with other family members.
- Don't use other people's eye cosmetics, particularly eye pencils and mascara.
- If your child gets pinkeye, keep her out of school until the infection clears up.

TIP 270

NUTRITIONAL AIDS FOR
NIGHT BLINDNESS

If you have night blindness, or difficulty seeing in dim light, try a daily 200 mg dose of bilberry *(Vaccinium myrtillus)*—reported to help improve microcirculation, the flow of blood in the vessels of the eye. Make sure you get sufficient vitamin A, which plays a key role in the eye's ability to adjust to different degrees of light.

TIP 271

BLACK EYE DO'S AND DON'TS

- Do apply something cold to the eye. An ice-cold compress will reduce swelling and constrict blood vessels, which will in turn stop the internal bleeding that causes the blue-black discoloration around the eye. Repeat for 5 to 10 minutes every hour for 24 hours or as long as swelling is present.
- Do use the homeopathic remedy *Ledom* or *Arnica,* both of which reduce swelling and speed healing.
- Don't blow your nose; it may rupture more blood vessels and cause greater discoloration.
- Don't force open an eyelid that is swollen shut; doing so could further injure the skin or the eye.
- Don't take aspirin, an anticoagulant. It will interfere with the clotting of the broken blood vessels around the eye, resulting in a bigger bruise.
- Do take acetaminophen to help reduce inflammation.
- Do see a doctor if you think your eyeball is damaged or if your vision is affected.

TIP *272*

GETTING THE RED OUT

If the whites of your eyes develop red lines, a sign of swollen blood vessels, you may simply need to get more sleep. Without sleep, eyes can become dry and red. Eyedrops that reduce redness should be used sparingly. Although they constrict blood vessels, which can make your eyes look whiter, they can also produce a rebound effect. A homeopathic remedy called Similisan # 1 Homeopathic Eyedrops is reputed to work without rebound. Or instead of using drops, try placing a cool, wet washcloth over your closed eyes. The cold will constrict the blood vessels and the water will moisten your eyes.

TIP *273*

COMFORT FOR DRY EYES

If your eyes often feel dry, hot, or scratchy, they probably do not have enough moisture. Aging is a common cause; tear production drops by about 60 percent from age 18 to age 65. Other contributing factors to dry eyes are low humidity, smoke, and medications such as antihistamines, decongestants, and birth control pills. To help keep your eyes moist, try the following:

- Stop smoking and avoid smoke-filled rooms.
- Reduce your exposure to direct wind, air-conditioning, and hair dryers.
- Use a humidifier during the dry winter months to add humidity to your house and place of work.
- Use an over-the-counter artificial tear solution.
- If your eyes are driest in the morning, ask your ophthalmologist about using a lubricating ointment at bedtime.
- Use homeopathic eyedrops.

TIP 274

TREAT A STY WITH WARMTH

To relieve the pain and inflammation of a sty—a red, tender swelling near the edge of the eyelid—apply a warm compress to the affected eye for 10 to 15 minutes four times daily for several days. Be sure to close your eye while you apply the compress. The heat of the compress will also help the sty ripen faster. When the sty comes to a head, continue applying warm compresses to relieve pressure and promote rupture. Never squeeze the sty; let it burst on its own.

TIP 275

STAVING OFF STIES

If you get recurring sties, try this preventive measure: Cleanse the outside of your eyelids daily. Put a few drops of very mild baby shampoo into a teacup of warm water and stir. Keeping your eyes closed, use a cotton swab to gently brush the mixture over your eyelids once a day.

TIP 276

REMOVING EARWAX

To remove earwax without damaging your ear, try this cleaning method: Warm 1 tbsp of hydrogen peroxide by setting the jar in a sinkful of hot water for a few minutes. Tilt your head to the side and put a dropperful of the warmed liquid in your blocked ear. Let it remain there for three minutes. Then tilt your head the other way and let the hydrogen peroxide run out onto a towel or tissue. The wax should be soft enough to wipe away with a piece of cotton. Repeat if necessary.

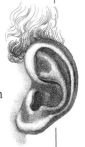

TIP *277*

HEALING HERBS FOR EAR INFECTIONS

The following herbs may help heal otitis media, an infection of the middle ear that is the most common cause of earaches.

- **Garlic** *(Allium sativum)* has been shown to act as a natural antibiotic. Put 1 to 3 drops of garlic oil in your ear three times daily.
- **Ginger** *(Zingiber officinale)* is considered another natural antibiotic. Take as a tincture or drink as a tea. *Tea: Put 1 tbsp of the fresh root in 1 cup boiling water; let simmer for 10 minutes. Drink several times a day.*
- **Echinacea** *(Echinacea* spp.) and **goldenseal** *(Hydrastis canadensis)* have anti-inflammatory properties. You can take either herb as a tincture or as a tea. *Tea: Pour a cup of boiling water over 1 to 2 tsp of dried echinacea; let seep for 10 to 15 minutes. Drink three times a day.*

ECHINACEA

TIP *278*

YOGA FOR HEARING LOSS

The Half Shoulder Stand and Fish positions may help some forms of hearing loss by increasing the circulation of blood to the ears.

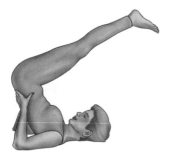

Half Shoulder Stand
Lie on your back, hands at your sides. Lift both legs until they are at a right angle to your back. Supporting your hips with your hands, inhale and extend your legs at the angle shown.

TIP *279*

A PRESSURE POINT THAT MAY IMPROVE HEARING

To enhance hearing, try applying pressure to the acupressure point known as Gall Bladder 2.

Gall Bladder 2
Open your mouth and, feeling along the jawbone, locate the depression directly in front of your ears. Place the tips of your middle fingers about one-half inch below the base of the depression. Close your mouth and press steadily on the point.

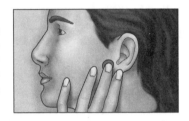

TIP *280*

BLOW-DRY YOUR EARS

If you are prone to recurrent bouts of swimmer's ear, an infection of the outer ear canal also known as otitis externa, try blow-drying your ears each time you shower or swim. Set the hair dryer on low and hold it about a foot from your ear. Let air blow into each of your ears for at least 30 seconds. The air will dry your ears, eliminating the moist environment that bacteria and fungi—the causes of swimmer's ear—find so hospitable.

TIP *281*

PREVENTIVE SOLUTIONS FOR SWIMMER'S EAR

Isopropyl alcohol and white vinegar help kill germs and dry the ears—and thus can help prevent swimmer's ear. After swimming or showering, tilt your head and put a few drops of either of these solutions—or a mixture of the two—into each ear. Wiggle the outside of your ear to help the solution get to the bottom of the ear canal; then tilt your head and let the liquid drain out.

TIP *282*

HERBAL DROPS
FOR SWIMMER'S EAR

Mullein *(Verbascum thapsus)* oil, which has anti-inflammatory properties, may help soothe and heal an inflamed ear canal. Put 1 to 3 drops in the infected ear every three hours. Garlic *(allium sativum)* may also help heal a swimmer's ear infection.

Ear drops: Combine equal parts garlic juice, glycerin, and a carrier oil, such as olive or sweet almond; put 1 to 3 drops in the infected ear every three hours.

MULLEIN

TIP *283*

RING OUT THAT
RINGING IN YOUR EARS

If you have tinnitus, the sensation of hearing ringing, buzzing, hissing, chirping, whistling or other sounds either intermittently or continuously through the day and night, try these remedies:

- Avoid alcohol, smoking, caffeine, salt, and aspirin; they can aggravate tinnitus and make the noises worse.
- Avoid loud noises, which can also worsen tinnitus.
- If you have trouble sleeping because of the noise in your ears, try turning on a radio, which can mask the unwanted sound with soothing music. Or record a "white noise" tape, such as the sound of running water, and play it whenever you need relief.
- Exercise regularly. It will increase blood circulation to the head and perhaps lessen the severity of the noises.
- Take supplements of B complex (50 mg) and zinc (22 mg) daily; deficiencies of either of these can lead to ringing in the ears.

TIP *284*

EARRING ALLERGIES

If your ear lobes develop an itchy, inflamed rash, you may be allergic to the nickel in your earrings. Remove the earrings at once and bathe your lobes with hydrogen peroxide. You may also want to apply calendula *(Calendula officinalis)* ointment to the infected areas three times a day. Once the infection has cleared up, wear only high-grade gold or pure silver earrings. Or you can try covering the backs of troublesome earrings with a barrier layer of clear nail polish.

TIP *285*

HOMEMADE NASAL SPRAY

To help thin nasal mucus caused by a cold, allergy or other condition, try this simple saline solution: Mix a teaspoon of table salt and a teaspoon of baking soda in a quart of water. Whenever you need to flush away excess mucus, tilt your head back and spray a small amount of the solution into each nostril. You'll have to buy a small spray bottle; try a well-stocked pharmacy.

TIP *286*

NEVER STIFLE A SNEEZE

If you repress a sneeze, you could force mucus into the middle ear or sinuses and cause an infection. In extreme cases, you could burst an eardrum from backed-up air pressure. So when you get the urge to sneeze—go for it. Be sure, however, to cover your mouth and nose to keep your germs from spreading to others.

TIP *287*

STEAM OPEN A STUFFY NOSE

Inhaling steam can help clear nasal passages. Take a hot bath or shower. Or drink anything hot from a cup, such as tea with ginger or lemon, or chicken soup. A humidifier can also help unclog a stuffy nose. For an extra effect, add essential oils of eucalyptus *(Eucalyptus globulus)*, tea tree *(Melaleuca* spp.), rosemary *(Rosmarinus officinalis)*, or peppermint *(Mentha piperita)* to the water in the humidifier during the day, and use the essential oil of lavender *(Lavandula officinalis)* in the evening. The lavender will also enhance your sleep.

LAVENDER

TIP *288*

HOMEMADE DECONGESTANT

When hay fever has clogged your nose, make your own decongestant by boiling grapefruit, orange, or lemon peels, including the pith, in water mixed with honey until the peels are spongy, stirring occasionally. Be careful not to overcook: You don't want candied fruit. Eat one piece when symptoms start and one piece each evening at bedtime during hay fever season. Substances in the peel and white rind act as anti-inflammatory agents and will dry mucous membranes.

TIP *289*

HERBAL ANTIBIOTICS

Several herbs have antimicrobial properties that can help fight the infection causing a sore throat. At the first sign of soreness, eat three raw cloves of garlic *(Allium sativum)* a day. If garlic odor becomes a problem, try four garlic oil capsules instead. Gylcerated tinctures of either goldenseal *(Hydrastis canadensis)* or echinacea *(Echinacea* spp.) may also be effective; take 15 drops twice a day to speed healing.

TIP *290*

HOMEMADE GARGLES

To relieve a sore throat, try any of these gargles:

- **Salt water:** *Mix ½ tsp salt in 8 oz warm water.*
- **Lemon:** *Mix the juice of one lemon in 8 oz warm water.*
- **Apple cider vinegar:** *Mix 2 tsp vinegar in 1 cup warm water.*
- **Cayenne pepper:** *Mix the juice of half a lemon, 1 tbsp salt, and ¼ tsp cayenne pepper (or more if you can tolerate it) in ½ cup warm water. The cayenne pepper temporarily reduces the amount of pain-causing chemicals produced by nerve endings in the throat.*

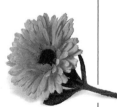

CAYENNE PEPPER

- **Calendula:** *Mix 1 part calendula (Calendula officinalis) with 1 part water and gargle every hour or so.*

CALENDULA

TIP*291*

TOOTHBRUSHES
DON'T LAST FOREVER

Bacteria can collect on the bristles of your toothbrush and lead to a throat infection. If you tend to get recurrent sore throats, you should replace your toothbrush every month. Also, be sure to toss an old toothbrush once you've recovered from a sore throat to avoid reinfecting yourself. And never share a toothbrush with someone else.

TIP*292*

TRY EUCALYPTUS-CYPRESS LOTION

To ease the discomfort of a sore throat, massage your throat and chest with a lotion made with 2 drops each of eucalyptus *(Eucalyptus globulus)* and cypress in 2 tsp of a carrier oil such as vegetable or almond oil. Rubbing the lotion into your skin will help increase blood circulation and improve fluid drainage in sore areas.

TIP*293*

USE A THROAT POULTICE

To help relieve the pain of a sore throat, try a warm chamomile poultice.

Poultice: Mix 1 tbsp dried chamomile flowers into 1 or 2 cups boiling water; steep for five minutes, then strain. Soak a clean cloth or towel in the tea, wring it out, then apply to your throat. Remove the cloth when it becomes cold. Repeat as often as necessary.

CHAMOMILE

TIP 294

ACT QUICKLY
TO FIGHT THE INFECTION

At the first sign of sore throat, take 1,000 to 3,000 mg of vitamin C daily to help fight the cold or other viral infection causing it. You may also wish to eat three raw cloves of garlic a day. Garlic *(Allium sativum)* is a natural antibiotic and antiseptic. If garlic odor becomes a problem, try four garlic oil capsules instead. Also, zinc lozenges are very good for sore throats.

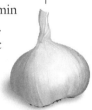

GARLIC

TIP 295

LARYNGITIS?
DON'T EVEN WHISPER

Whispering is not a good idea when you have laryngitis. In fact, whispering forces you to use your vocal cords in a way that is just as harmful as shouting. To regain your voice, your best bet is to stay completely quiet. Keep your larynx wet by drinking 8 to 10 glasses of water daily and by inhaling steam from a bowl or sink of steaming water or a cup of ginger tea for 5 minutes several times a day.

Joints, Bones, and Muscles

TIP *296*

HERBAL REMEDIES
FOR PAINFUL JOINTS

To relieve the pain of arthritis or bursitis, many herbalists recommend a 5 ml tincture made from 2 parts willow *(Salix* spp.) bark and 1 part each of black cohosh *(Cimicifuga racemosa)* and nettle *(Urtica dioica).* To relieve muscle tension, herbalists recommend rubbing the affected area with a liniment made from a tincture of lobelia *(Lobelia inflata)* and cramp *(Viburnum opulus)* bark. The Chinese herbal formula Du Huo Ji Sheng Wan may also help for some types of arthritis. Consult an experienced herbalist for specific treatment.

NETTLE

TIP *297*

LEARN THE ABCS
FOR ARTHRITIS

Vitamin therapy may be helpful in relieving some of your arthritic symptoms. Beta carotene (vitamin A) has an antioxidant effect on cells, neutralizing destructive molecules called free radicals that may play a part in the degeneration of joint tissue. Vitamins C, B_6, and E, as well as zinc, are thought to help repair damaged joint tissue. Niacin (vitamin B_3) may also be helpful, although excessive use may aggravate liver problems. If you are taking aspirin regularly to relieve arthritic pain, you also need to make sure you are getting enough vitamin C. Aspirin can deplete the body's vitamin C balance. Always take vitamin supplements under professional guidance, since overdoses of some vitamin compounds can have side effects or undesirable interactions with drugs.

TIP*298*

VITAMIN D
FOR YOUR KNEES

Recent research suggests that elderly people with osteoarthritis of the knee can control the progression of the disease by doubling their vitamin D intake from 200 (the current Recommended Dietary Allowance) to 400 units a day. Scientists believe that vitamin D plays an essential role in keeping cartilage and bone in the knee joint from degenerating. If you have been diagnosed with osteoarthritis, try including more vitamin D-rich foods in your diet, such as milk, eggs, fortified cereals, and fatty fish. Or talk to your doctor about taking vitamin D supplements. And be sure to get daily exposure to sunlight, which the body needs to properly synthesize vitamin D.

TIP*299*

GET IN THE WATER

If you have arthritis, head for the pool. Swimming and other water exercise, preferably in a heated pool, may be the key to helping you pursue a more active and less painful life. With the water supporting your body and reducing the stress of gravity, you will be able to work on expanding the movement of your affected joints and improving your muscle strength.

TIP *300*

HOMEOPATHIC REMEDIES FOR ARTHRITIS

You may find the following homeopathic ingredients helpful in relieving your arthritis symptoms.

- *Bryonia* may help ease arthritic pain that is aggravated by motion, touch, or entering a warm room.
- *Pulsatilla* may help if the pain tends to move from joint to joint and does not settle in one area.
- *Silica* may help if you have osteoarthritis or another form of arthritis that has developed slowly over a long period of time.
- *Colchicum* may help ease arthritic pain aggravated by cold and damp weather.

These ingredients are usually prescribed as part of a broader constitutional remedy. Consult a trained homeopathic practitioner for the remedy that will work best for you.

TIP *301*

A HOT OINTMENT FOR ARTHRITIS

For temporary relief of osteoarthritis and rheumatoid arthritis pain, try an over-the-counter ointment made with cayenne *(Capsicum annuum* var. *annuum)*. Capsicum, the active ingredient in cayenne, is believed to increase blood flow to joint tissues, thereby reducing inflammation. Because cayenne ointment feels very hot when rubbed onto the skin, it should be used for only short periods.

CAYENNE

TIP *302*

USE YOGA TO LOOSEN JOINTS

Daily yoga practice may help loosen stiff, arthritic joints. Try the exercises shown here for painful joints in your hands, hips and back.

Spider

Press your fingertips together firmly, holding your palms two to three inches apart. Then push your palms toward each other (near right) and with your fingertips still together move them apart (far right). Relax, then repeat the push-up motion.

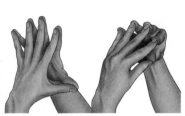

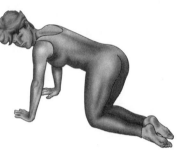

C

On your hands and knees, exhale and swing your head and buttocks as far to the left as you can. Inhale as you slowly straighten your back, and then do the same movement to the right. Do this 10 times.

TIP *303*

APPLY HEAT TO SORE JOINTS

For immediate relief from most kinds of joint pain, apply dry heat from a heating pad or moist heat in the form of a hot bath or a hot-water bottle wrapped in a towel. If the joint appears inflamed and swollen, however, apply a cold pack instead for 10 to 15 minutes every hour until you notice improvement; then you can switch to heat to speed healing.

TIP *304*

GINGER ROOT OVER CASTOR OIL

A commonly recommended natural treatment for the pain of bursitis is to apply a castor-oil pack. Even better, and far less messy, is the ginger-root *(Zingiber officinale)* variety. To make the pack, simmer 2 tbsp chopped ginger in 3 cups water for 20 minutes, then soak a piece of white cotton or wool flannel in the water, and squeeze out the excess. Place the pack over the affected area for 5 to 7 minutes, and repeat 3 to 4 times a day. Between applications, store the pack in a pot in the refrigerator. You can reheat and reuse the pack for up to three days before discarding.

GINGER

TIP *305*

A RESCUE REMEDY
FOR BURSITIS

To reduce the inflammation of bursitis, try the Bach flower remedy known as Rescue Remedy. Apply it in cream form to the painful joint three or four times a day. Rescue Remedy is a combination of five other flower-essence remedies: Cherry Plum, Clematis, Impatiens, Rock Rose, and Star-of-Bethlehem.

TIP *306*

GET OFF YOUR HIGH HEELS

Your best bet for preventing bunions, those knobby, painful protrusions at the base of the big toe, is to wear shoes that fit properly. Avoid shoes that cramp or pinch your toes. Women should be wary of high-heeled, pointed shoes styled more for fashion than for comfort and good support. Shoes that fit badly can force your bones to gradually assume an unnatural shape, leading not only to the formation of a painful bunion (or a bunionette on the little toe), but also to bursitis in other areas of the foot.

TIP *307*

THROW RICE AT A SORE JOINT

For a speedier recovery from a sprain, strain, or other muscle or joint injury, start the following four-point RICE program as soon as the injury occurs.

1. **R**est the sore joint.
2. **I**ce the joint for 10 to 15 minutes every hour. You can use a bag of frozen vegetables if no ice pack is handy.
3. **C**ompress the area by wrapping it snugly, but not painfully tight, in a sports bandage.
4. **E**levate the joint by putting your ankle on a footstool or your elbow on a chairside table. This will help reduce blood pressure in the injured area.

TIP *308*

WHEN THE TENDON STAYS SORE

If you suffer from a chronic case of tendinitis, apply alternating hot and cold compresses to the sore area. Soak one washcloth in hot water and another in cold. Wring out the warm cloth and place it over the affected area for three minutes; follow with the cold cloth for 30 seconds. Alternate them two more times, finishing with the cold cloth. Do this once or twice a day, as needed.

TIP *309*

BUILD BULK

When a tendon becomes sore, the muscles around it weaken, which leaves the tendon very susceptible to reinjury. So once your tendinitis heals, you should devise a weightlifting program for yourself that gradually rebuilds the weakened muscles. Don't overdo it, however; putting too much strain on the muscles too soon may cause the tendon to become inflamed again.

TIP 310

PREVENTING
NIGHTTIME LEG CRAMPS

If the calves of your legs tend to cramp at night while you're lying in bed, try these spasm-prevention tips:

- Sleep on your side, and try not to point your toes. Most nocturnal leg cramps are caused by sudden toe-pointing, which contracts the calf muscles.
- Avoid tucking in your sheets and blankets too tightly so your toes will have plenty of wiggle room.
- Do gentle stretching exercises before going to bed.

To stop a calf cramp that strikes while you're lying in bed, flex your foot by pointing your toes up toward your shin. Or grab the toes and ball of your foot and gently pull them toward your knee.

TIP 311

TAKE GINKGO FOR LEG SPASMS

Gingko *(Ginkgo biloba)* tea may help improve circulation and relieve leg spasms. Or take 15 drops of ginkgo tincture or two capsules twice a day.

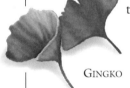

Tea: *Pour a cup of boiling water onto 2 tsp of the dried herb and steep for 15 to 20 minutes; drink three times a day.*

GINGKO

TIP 312

THE PINEAPPLE TREATMENT

To reduce inflammation of tendons and other soft body tissues, some herbalists recommend bromelain, an enzyme found in pineapples. Bromelain supplements can be found in most health food stores. Take as directed; some preparations recommend taking with food, others before or after eating.

TIP *313*

NOT JUST FOR
TENNIS PLAYERS

Anyone who works with his or her hands—house painters, carpenters, and seamstresses, for example—can develop tennis elbow, or recurring pain on the outside of the upper forearm just below the bend of the elbow. If you work a lot with your hands, you may wish to take these precautionary measures:

- Lift objects with your palm facing your body.
- Try strengthening exercises with hand weights. With your elbow cocked and your palm down, repeatedly bend your wrist. Stop if you feel any pain.
- Stretch relevant muscles before beginning a possibly stressful activity by grasping the top part of your fingers and gently but firmly pulling them back toward your body. Keep your arm fully extended and your palm facing outward.

TIP *314*

HERBAL OILS
FOR TENDER MUSCLES

Mix together any of the following essential oils with a carrier oil such as sweet almond, apricot kernel, or jojoba oil, and massage the blend on sore, tender muscles and joints to increase blood flow and speed healing.

- Prickly ash *(Zanthoxylum americanum)*
- Lavender *(Lavandula officinalis)*
- Safflower *(Carthamus tinctorius)*
- Eucalyptus *(Eucalyptus globulus)*
- Ginger *(Zingiber officinale)*

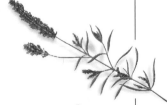

LAVENDER

TIP *315*

SUPPLEMENTS FOR
STRAINS AND SPRAINS

Although most sprained joints or strained muscles will heal with rest, research suggests you can help speed the process with various vitamin supplements. If your doctor approves, take daily supplements of vitamin C (1,000 mg), vitamin A (10,000 IU), zinc (up to 60 mg), vitamin E (400 IU), and selenium (50 mcg).

TIP *316*

DO HOURLY HAND EXERCISES

If you have a job or hobby that calls for repetitive hand or finger work, be sure to take breaks and exercise your hands and wrists every hour to avoid the painful and disabling injury known as carpal tunnel syndrome. Here are three quick hand routines:

1. Open and close your fist a dozen times or more.
2. With palms facing each other, press your fingertips together 20 times, rest, then repeat.
3. Holding your hands over your head, rotate them at the wrists clockwise for 20 seconds, then do the same exercise counterclockwise.

TIP *317*

GET THE B_6 BENEFIT

If you are suffering from carpal tunnel syndrome, you may want to up your intake of Vitamin B_6. Research has shown that vitamin B_6 can help relieve the symptoms of the syndrome, perhaps by healing nerve inflammation and enhancing blood circulation. Start with 50 mg a day, or try a vitamin B complex supplement; symptoms should ease within a month to six weeks. You may also want to reduce your protein intake, as a high-protein diet can inhibit the absorption of B_6.

TIP *318*

HOT VINEGAR

For tendinitis, sprains, strains, and other forms of joint pain, try a hot vinegar pack: Heat equal parts vinegar and water, then soak a towel in the mixture. Wring it out and apply it to the affected area for five minutes. Remove it, then apply a cold one for five minutes. Cover with wool. Repeat these hot-cold applications three times, finishing with cold.

TIP *319*

REFLEXOLOGY RELIEF
FOR A GROIN PULL

To ease the pain and discomfort of a groin pull, try the following reflexology technique.

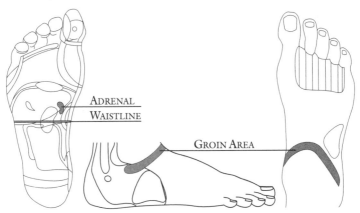

ADRENAL
WAISTLINE
GROIN AREA

Holding your foot straight back, walk your left index finger from one side of the groin area to the other; walk back with your right finger. Repeat several times. Then push the big toe back and walk your thumb along the inside of the main tendon on the bottom of your foot from the waistline area to the adrenal area.

TIP 320

STRETCHES TO PROTECT
YOUR HAMSTRINGS

Before starting your favorite sport or physical activity, particularly those that put heavy demands on your legs, take a few minutes to warm up your hamstring muscles along the back of your thighs. The following two exercises are especially good for conditioning and strengthening the hamstrings.

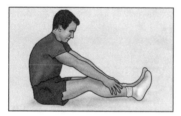

Sit on the floor with your legs extended and slightly bent at the knees, keeping your back as straight as possible. Slowly bend from the hips and reach down your legs as far as you can, without forcing the stretch. Hold in place for 15 seconds.

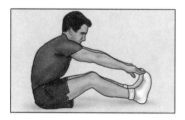

Without changing your position, reach toward your feet and try to touch your toes with your fingertips. Hold this position for 15 seconds, then slowly relax the stretch and sit back. Rest for 20 seconds, then repeat the exercise. Do 8 to 10 times.

TIP 321

GOT GOUT? GO VEGGIE

Gout is uncommon among vegetarians, most likely because their meatless diet is usually lower in purines, a substance that can lead to abnormally high levels of uric acid in the bloodstream—the cause of gout. So if you have a hereditary predisposition to gout, you may want to reduce or eliminate your intake of fish, meat, and poultry. Animal products that have particularly high levels of purines in them include organ meats, such as liver, sweetbreads, and kidneys, and shellfish and certain kinds of preserved fish, including sardines, herring, and anchovies.

TIP 322

EAT CHERRIES

Some people report that eating cherries helps relieve gout. To try
the cherry cure, eat up to 8 oz of sweet or sour cherries a day.
The fruit can be either fresh or canned. Or, if you prefer,
take 1 tbsp of cherry concentrate daily.

TIP 323

TRY CALCIUM SUPPLEMENTS

If you have difficulty getting enough calcium through your diet,
you may want to take calcium supplements. Calcium supplements
are available in many forms, but chelated forms, such as calcium
citrate and calcium gluconate, appear to be more effective at reducing bone loss. Avoid using dolomite or bone meal as calcium
supplements or taking calcium carbonate supplements labeled
"oyster shell," as they may contain lead and other toxic metals.

TIP 324

PUT YOUR SUPPLEMENT
TO THE TEST

Some calcium supplements are better absorbed into the body
than others. To determine whether the calcium in your supplement tablets is easily absorbed by your body, try this test:

*Calcium test: Drop a tablet into 6 oz of vinegar at room
temperature. Stir every two to three minutes. The tablet
should disintegrate within 30 minutes. If it does not, try
another kind.*

TIP 325

DON'T FORGET VITAMIN D

To help your body absorb calcium, you need adequate amounts of vitamin D in your diet. Most people easily get enough vitamin D by eating a normal diet and spending 10 to 15 minutes out in the sun several times a week. Sunlight activates a compound in the skin that the kidneys and liver convert into a usable form of vitamin D. As you age, however, your body gets less adept at manufacturing vitamin D from sunlight. By the age of 60, if you want to help keep your bones strong, you need to eat more vitamin D-rich foods or take a daily supplement. Good food sources include milk fortified with vitamin D, fortified breakfast cereals, egg yolks, canned sardines, canned tuna, saltwater fish, and liver. If you decide to try supplements, don't take more than 400 IUs daily without consulting your doctor; an overdose of vitamin D can be dangerous.

TIP 326

ADD VINEGAR
TO YOUR SOUP STOCK

When making soup stock from bones, add a little vinegar to the water. The vinegar will dissolve some of the calcium out of the bones, for a calcium-fortified soup. A pint of the stock can contain as much as 1,000 mg of calcium.

TIP 327

PRESSURE POINT
FOR NECK STRESS

To reduce neck muscle stress that may cause head or back pain, try applying pressure to the acupressure point known as Gall Bladder 20.

Gall Bladder 20
Place the tips of your middle fingers in the hollows at the base of your skull, about two inches apart on either side of the spine. Press firmly.

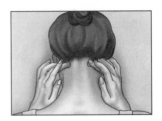

TIP 328

THE BEST TLC FOR TMJ

Biofeedback, a technique that uses special computerized equipment to translate muscle tension into audible signals, is considered the most effective mind/body treatment for temporomandibular joint syndrome, or TMJ. Using electrical readings from the muscle that moves your jaw, a biofeedback practitioner can train you to control the tension in that area of your face. Once you learn the technique, you can self-administer it. Consult an experienced biofeedback practitioner.

TIP 329

WEAR A MOUTH GUARD TO BED

If your TMJ is caused by bruxism, or grinding your teeth at night, you may want to consider wearing a mouth guard while you sleep. Your dentist can fit you with a bite guard. Or you can purchase a sports mouth guard—the kind worn by football and hockey players—at a sporting goods store.

TIP *330*

TRY ACUPUNCTURE
FOR BACK PROBLEMS

If you are troubled by back problems, you may want to give acupuncture a try. In the hands of a trained acupuncturist, needle therapy not only relieves immediate or chronic back pain, but also redirects energy flow and provides balance throughout the body. Acupuncture involves inserting needles into points in specific muscles and the ear to relieve what are considered in Chinese medicine to be blockages in the energy channels associated with back pain. Acute problems usually involve one to four sessions, while chronic pain problems typically require 12 or more treatments.

TIP *331*

RELAX YOUR BACK WITH BIOFEEDBACK

Biofeedback therapy is another worthwhile option for back problems. It uses special computerized equipment to translate muscle tension into audible signals. Under the guidance of a trained biofeedback practitioner, you will learn how to slow the signals and relax your back muscles. Or, if you prefer, you could try guided imagery treatments, which offer similar results without the use of electronic equipment.

TIP *332*

HOMEOPATHY FOR BACK PAIN

Several over-the-counter homeopathic remedies are reported to help nonspecific back problems. These include *Arnica* for bruised or sore muscles, *Bryonia* and *Rhus toxicodendron* for sharp pain that worsens when you move, and *Ruta* for persistent backache.

TIP*333*

TEST YOUR POSTURE

The most important preventive measure for lower back pain is practicing good posture. To analyze your posture, stand with your heels against a wall. Your calves, buttocks, shoulders, and the back of your head should touch the wall, and you should be able to slip your hand behind the small of your back. Then step forward and stand normally: If your posture changes, correct it right away. If your posture problems persist, you may wish to see an Alexander technique or Feldenkrais method practitioner, who can help you learn how to realign your body.

TIP*334*

CHECK OUT YOUR CHAIR

The source of your back problem may be in the chair in which you sit for much of the day. So size up your seat: A good chair bottom supports your hips but doesn't touch the backs of your knees. Your chair back should be set at an angle of about 10 degrees and should cradle the small of your back comfortably; if necessary, use a wedge-shaped cushion or lumbar pad. Your feet should rest flat on the floor. Your forearms should rest on your desk or work surface, with your elbows almost at a right angle.

TIP 335

LIFT WITH YOUR LEGS

To protect your back, let your leg muscles, not your back muscles, do the lifting when you have to pick up heavy objects. Here's how: Squat with your legs, keep your back straight and upright as you grasp the object, and stand upright again. You may also find a nonprescription back brace useful in preventing back strain, primarily because it won't let you bend over at the waist. But use a back brace sparingly: Long-term use can make you dependent on it and may eventually lead to weaker—not stronger—back muscles.

TIP 336

PUT YOUR BACK IN
THE HANDS OF A CHIROPRACTOR

If you are looking for a drug-free treatment option for back pain, you may want to consult an experienced chiropractor. Chiropractic spinal manipulation has been recognized by the U.S. Agency for Health Care Policy and Research as an effective therapy for acute low-back pain. The manipulation corrects subluxations, or misaligned vertebrae, which may be responsible for problems anywhere along the spine. Many chiropractors combine spinal manipulation with muscle massage, ultrasound stimulation of deep tissue, nutritional recommendations, and exercise.

TIP 337

REGAIN MOBILITY

Massage of the muscles along both sides of the spine helps relieve tension and restore mobility, especially in areas that feel tight or hard. To avoid potential damage to the spinal cord, visit a trained physical therapist or massage therapist who will be careful not to exert direct pressure on the vertebrae themselves.

TIP 338

HERBAL RELIEF

For general pain relief, drink infusions of white willow *(Salix alba)* or vervain *(Verbena officinalis)*. For inflammation, try teas brewed from yarrow *(Achillea millefolium)*, cramp *(Viburnum opulus)*, or white willow. Valerian *(Valeriana officinalis)*, available as a tincture and in capsules, is particularly recommended as a muscle relaxant and sedative.

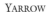

YARROW

TIP 339

PRESS AWAY LOWER-BACK PAIN

To relieve lower-back pain, apply 60 seconds of thumb pressure on either side of the spine, just above the top of the pelvic bone. Then massage this point, as well as at the hip and knee joint.

TIP *340*

YOGA STRETCHES
FOR THE LOWER BACK

The following yoga exercises will help stretch and strengthen the muscles of your lower back, thus helping to prevent disk and other back problems.

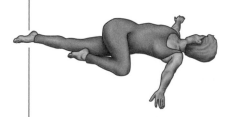

Knee Down Twist

Lie on your back with your arms out. Inhale and place your right foot on your left knee. Exhale, then turn your head to the right and bring your right knee toward the floor to your left. Release slowly, then repeat on the other side.

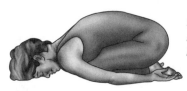

Child

Sit on your heels, knees together. With your arms at your sides, palms up, bend from the hips and extend your upper body over your knees, bringing your forehead toward the floor. Then slowly sit up.

TIP *341*

OSTEOPATHY

Try spinal manipulation, given by an osteopath, a chiropractor, or a physical therapist, for back-pain relief. Osteopathic treatment combines drug therapy with spinal manipulation or traction, followed by physical therapy or exercise.

TIP *342*

SELF-MASSAGE FOR SCIATICA

The painful condition called sciatica occurs when the sciatic nerve at the base of the spine is compressed, causing pain to radiate through the buttocks and down the back of the thigh. To ease the pain, try this self-massage technique: Lie on your back with knees bent; relax for several minutes; take a sock containing two soft rubber balls and position them on either side of your spine in the small of your back; allow your body weight to sink into the floor, over the balls. Remove the balls and relax for a few more minutes. Follow the same procedure for your buttocks. (If you have disk problems, check with your doctor before trying this.)

TIP *343*

BACKACHE RELIEF DURING PREGNANCY

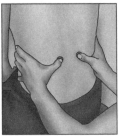

Bladder 23
This point site is level with the space between the second and third lumbar vertebrae. Find BL 23 by aligning your thumbs or fingers about an inch outward from either side of the spine, just behind the navel, then press inward.

To alleviate backache due to pregnancy, try the following:

• Stimulate acupressure point Bladder 23 *(left)*. Or rub the same area vigorously enough with the back of your hand to create heat.

• Sit up straight, and whenever possible, sit with your legs elevated.

• Don't stand for long periods and don't stretch to reach high places.

• Sit backward on a straight chair. Lean over the back with your head resting on your crossed arms. Have a partner massage your back with long strokes, working upward and outward from the lower back, avoiding pressure on the spine.

Your Healthy Heart

TIP 344

HAWTHORN TEA

To strengthen arteries and tone the heart, herbalists recommend hawthorn *(Crataegus laevigata)*. You can drink the herb as a tea by brewing its flowers, leaves, and berries, or take it in extract or tincture form. But if you have high blood pressure or suspect you might, consult your doctor first.

HAWTHORN

TIP 345

STEER CLEAR OF
SMOKE AND SMOG

Certain air pollutants, particularly carbon monoxide, are known to aggravate and intensify angina. To avoid carbon monoxide, steer clear of tobacco smoke and stay inside on heavy smog days.

TIP 346

WHAT'S YOUR SHAPE?

Studies have shown that people who are apple-shaped—or who carry most of their fat around their stomach—are at a greater risk of developing heart disease than people whose bodies are pear-shaped, or whose fat tends to accumulate around their hips. So if you have an apple-shaped body, be especially vigilant about following a heart-healthy lifestyle.

TIP *347*

AN "A" FOR VITAMIN E

If you want to lower your risk of heart disease, up your daily intake of vitamin E. Research suggests that the vitamin helps keep arteries from thickening and also increases high-density lipoprotein (HDL) levels (often called the "good cholesterol")—and thus may help protect against heart attacks and stroke. Good food sources of vitamin E are fortified cereals, olive oil, nuts, sunflower-seed kernels, kale, wheat germ, dried apricots, sweet potatoes, and mangoes. (But if you have high blood pressure already, vitamin E can aggravate it; check with your doctor.)

TIP *348*

S-L-O-W D-O-W-N

One of the keys to preventing and treating heart disease is learning how to relax. Relaxation reduces stress, and stress has been identified as a probable risk factor for heart disease. Some relaxation techniques that have proved beneficial are meditation, yoga, progressive relaxation, prayer, and biofeedback training. Find a relaxation program that you enjoy and incorporate it into your daily routine.

TIP *349*

WATCH YOUR WEIGHT

To stabilize both blood pressure and cholesterol levels, keep your weight in check. Even modest drops of excess poundage have been shown to be beneficial.

TIP *350*

THE MEAT OF THE MATTER

Vegetarians—particularly strict vegetarians called vegans who exclude dairy products and eggs as well as all meats from their diet—generally have a lower risk of heart disease than meat-eaters, because their diets contain less fat and cholesterol. To become a vegetarian, you don't have to give up meat "cold turkey." Start by eliminating meat from your diet one day a week, then two days a week, and so on, until you no longer miss it at the table.

TIP *351*

THE SLANT ON SLEEPING ASLANT

Some doctors recommend that to help eliminate nighttime angina attacks, you sleep on a tilted bed. By positioning yourself with your head several inches higher than your feet, more blood will pool in your legs—and less will try to painfully force its way through your clogged arteries. But other practitioners point out that less blood to your heart ultimately weakens it. Best advice: Talk over this strategy with your physician.

TIP *352*

DON'T FORGET YOUR FOLIC ACID

Research suggests that people whose diets are rich in folic acid (vitamin B_9) are less likely to die of heart disease than those whose diets lack it. Folic acid helps reduce blood levels of homocysteine, a compound that has been linked to an increased risk of heart attack and stroke. To make sure you're getting enough folic acid, try eating more dark leafy greens, orange juice, broccoli, peas, dried beans and fortified cereals.

TIP 353

EXPRESS YOURSELF

People who have a tendency to suppress their emotions when under stress—a personality trait known as "type D"—are at a greater risk of dying of heart disease than people who openly express their concerns and feelings. With the help of a trained therapist or a caring loved one, learn how to speak your mind in a positive and heart-healthy way.

TIP 354

CHOMP ON CELERY

If you have high blood pressure, try snacking on celery. For centuries, Chinese health practitioners have prescribed celery and celery oil to patients suffering from high blood pressure and other circulatory problems. Recent scientific research suggests why: A compound in the vegetable appears to relax the muscles in the lining of the arteries, thus allowing blood to flow more freely.

TIP 355

GO GUNG-HO ON GARLIC

Another great food for lowering blood pressure and cholesterol is garlic *(Allium sativum)*. Eating at least one whole clove a day, either raw or cooked in food, is best.

TIP *356*

HOMEOPATHY FOR ANGINA

To immediately relieve the pain of an acute angina attack, home-opaths recommend the following:

- *Cactus grandiflorus* if during the attack your chest feels like it's bound with an iron band.
- *Latrodectus mactans* if the pain is radiating down your left arm and you are having difficulty breathing.
- *Naja tripudians* if the pain is radiating up into the neck or shoulder and is accompanied by anxiety and coldness.

TIP *357*

AN AYURVEDIC AID

To reduce the frequency and severity of angina attacks, you may wish to try an Ayurvedic (Hindu) mixture of herbs and minerals known as Abana. Available in tablet form, Abana is typically prescribed for adults in an initial dosage of two tablets two or three times daily, then one tablet two or three times daily for maintenance. Consult an Ayurvedic practitioner for the specific dosage.

TIP *358*

A ROOT REMEDY

For the treatment of atherosclerosis, Chinese health practitioners recommend a number of herbs, including notoginseng *(Panax notoginseng)* root. (Its Chinese name is *tien chi.*) Consult a practitioner of Chinese medicine for exact mixtures and dosages.

TIP *359*

A LITTLE WINE IS FINE

Drinking a glass of red wine each day may offer you some protection against atherosclerosis and coronary artery disease. Studies suggest that flavonoids in grape skins, which give red wine its color and flavor, inhibit buildup of fatty deposits. But keep your wine consumption to a minimum; more than two ounces of alcohol per day can aggravate high blood pressure.

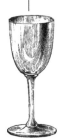

TIP *360*

DON'T OVERDO VITAMIN D

If you are taking vitamin supplements, make sure you stick near the Recommended Dietary Guidelines for vitamin D (200 IU, or 5 mcg, for adults). More than 400 IUs of vitamin D may actually speed up the formation of arterial plaques and the onset of atherosclerosis.

TIP *361*

PRESS FOR LOWER PRESSURE

To help regulate blood pressure, try applying pressure to the acupressure point known as Spleen 6.

Spleen 6
Measure four finger widths up from the top of the right inside anklebone. With your thumb, press near the edge of the shinbone. Repeat on the other leg. (Do not apply pressure to this point if you are pregnant.)

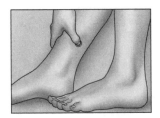

TIP *362*

GET MOVING

Regular aerobic workouts condition the heart and keep blood vessels dilated and working properly. Little wonder, then, that couch potatoes and other sedentary folks are two times more likely to develop heart disease than people who work out regularly. So get up and get moving. The best aerobic exercises are walking, running, swimming, cycling, skating, and cross-country skiing.

TIP *363*

AVOID AN IRON OVERLOAD

Do not take iron supplements unless blood tests indicate you have an iron deficiency and your doctor has advised you to take them. Although iron is essential for good health, too much of the mineral can lead to heart disease.

TIP *364*

DONATE BLOOD

The life you save when you donate blood may be your own. Bleeding is the body's natural way of ridding itself of iron, which at excess levels can increase your risk of heart disease. So when you give blood regularly, you may be ridding your body of surplus iron—and thus lowering your risk of heart disease.

TIP *365*

AN ASPIRIN A DAY

Talk to your doctor about taking an aspirin daily. Studies show that doses as low as 30 mg a day can significantly reduce the risk of heart attack, most likely by keeping blood clots from forming.

TIP 366

A LITTLE HELP
FROM YOUR FRIENDS

Stay in touch with friends and family. Reach out to others and build a community of caring people around you. Research has shown that people who live socially isolated lives are more vulnerable to heart disease.

TIP 367

BE A SODIUM SPY

Too much sodium—the key ingredient in salt—can cause high blood pressure in some people. If you are sodium-sensitive, you'll need to do more than put away your salt shaker. Excessive sodium is hidden in many processed and packaged foods. Read food labels carefully.

TIP 368

TRACK YOUR
BLOOD PRESSURE AT HOME

If you have high blood pressure, monitoring it every day with a home blood-pressure measuring device may be a good idea. Regular monitoring can let you know if your medication and self-help remedies for lowering your blood pressure are actually working. It can also help identify "office" hypertension—blood pressure that goes up simply because you're stressed out about being in a doctor's office. Take your blood pressure at about the same time every day to rule out natural daily fluctuations.

TIP*369*

SPEAK THE TRUTH

Studies have shown that lying can cause blood pressure to soar. Researchers speculate that when people are trying to deceive, their brains have to work extra hard, which requires more blood to flow to the brain—thus raising blood pressure. Lying also produces stress, another factor that sends blood pressure climbing. So speak from your heart; it may help protect it.

TIP*370*

SMOKING AND YOUR HEART

Kicking the nicotine habit is, without doubt, the best thing you can do for your heart and your health. People who smoke are more than twice as likely to suffer a heart attack than nonsmokers—and four times more likely to die from it within an hour. In all, smoking causes more than 200,000 deaths from cardiovascular disease in the United States each year. When you quit, your heart begins to benefit almost immediately. After two years of not smoking, much of your risk of heart disease will have disappeared. And within five to ten years, your risk will be the same as if you had never smoked.

TIP*371*

DRINK TEA

Tea contains catechin, a substance that has been shown to lower cholesterol. In one study, people with a high-cholesterol diet who drank tea regularly were able to keep their blood cholesterol levels within the normal range. Because of the way its leaves are processed, green tea, also known as Japanese or Chinese tea, contains more catechin than black tea.

TIP 372

THE CHOLESTEROL CUT-OFF

Although there is no magic number at which your cholesterol
level suddenly shifts from dangerous to safe, most experts
believe that you should aim to stay as low as possible below the
200 mg/ dl (milligrams of cholesterol per deciliter of blood)
level. Once cholesterol breeches the 220 level, the risk of heart
disease begins to rise rapidly.

TIP 373

CHOLESTEROL TEST
DO'S AND DON'TS

To ensure you get the most accurate results from your cholesterol
blood test, follow these precautions:

- Don't exercise before the test; physical exertion can
  increase your cholesterol levels by 10 to 15 percent.
- Don't eat anything for 12 hours beforehand; a recent meal can throw off your readings.
- Do be seated for the test; if you are standing or lying
  down when your blood is drawn, the concentration
  of lipoproteins in your blood may be affected.
- Do inform the person giving the test of any medications you are taking or recent illnesses you have had,
  as these can affect your cholesterol levels.

TIP 374

FROM THE SEA

Spirulina, a protein-rich type of algae, may help improve your
cholesterol profile. In daily doses of 1,400 mg, spirulina has
been shown to lower low-density lipoprotein (LDL) levels in
people with high blood pressure. Spirulina is available in powdered or tablet form.

TIP *375*

ORIENTAL OIL

Try preparing meals with lemongrass *(Cymbopogon citratus)* oil, a common flavoring in Oriental cooking. Research has shown that its regular use can reduce total cholesterol levels by more than 10 percent, perhaps by inhibiting the creation of cholesterol from dietary fats.

TIP *376*

CHARCOAL CARRYOUT

Often taken to relieve intestinal gas, activated charcoal has also been shown to reduce low-density lipoprotein (LDL) levels. In one study, people who took ¼ ounces of activated charcoal three times daily for four weeks experienced a 41 percent drop in their LDL levels. Researchers theorize that the charcoal hooks up with cholesterol molecules in the arteries and carries them safely out of the body.

TIP *377*

"C" IS FOR GOOD CHOLESTEROL

Consuming moderately high levels of vitamin C (around 300 mg daily) may help reduce your risk of heart disease. The vitamin has been shown effective in raising blood levels of protective high-density lipoproteins (HDLs). The foods richest in vitamin C are citrus fruits and dark leafy vegetables, such as broccoli, spinach and collard greens.

TIP*378*

THE CALCIUM-CHOLESTEROL CONNECTION

Calcium may help your heart as well as your bones. In one study, people who took 2 grams of calcium daily for a full year experienced a 25 percent reduction in their blood cholesterol levels.

TIP*379*

GRAZE

Eating smaller, more frequent meals throughout the day (without upping your total daily calories) may aid you in lowering your cholesterol. Here's why: When you eat a big meal, a large amount of insulin is released in your body. The insulin sets off the production of an enzyme, which in turn signals the liver to make more cholesterol. By eating smaller meals, therefore, you may limit the insulin release—and your cholesterol count.

TIP*380*

THE BUGS BUNNY APPROACH

Carrots have plenty of pectin, a fiber that helps carry cholesterol out of the digestive system before the cholesterol gets into the blood. Eating just two carrots a day may help lower your cholesterol by as much as 20 percent.

TIP*381*

A HOT TIP

Cook with cayenne *(Capsicum annuum* var. *annuum)* regularly and you'll have a recipe for a healthier heart. Cayenne acts as an all-around tonic for your circulatory system. It increases blood flow from the heart, lowers blood pressure, thins the blood, and helps clear clogged arteries.

CAYENNE

TIP*382*

SOY—BUT NOT THE OIL

Soybeans are rich in isoflavones, which have been shown to lower cholesterol levels and thus the risk of heart disease. Soybeans are made into a variety of food products, including tofu, tempeh and miso, which are now sold in most grocery stores. Cooking with soy oil, however, will not help reduce your cholesterol as it does not contain isoflavones.

TIP*383*

ALL IN THE FAMILY

Know your family's heart disease history. If any male in your family died suddenly or had a heart attack before the age of 55 or any female before the age of 65, you should take yourself and that information to a cardiologist well before you reach those ages. You may have inherited a predisposition to heart disease.

TIP*384*

TREAT YOUR HEART GINGERLY

Ginger *(Zingiber officinale)* has been shown to help prevent heart disease and strokes by reducing internal blood clotting and lowering blood pressure. You can add fresh or dried ginger to your food or take the herb in liquid extract, tablet, or capsule form. Ginger also makes a delicious tea.

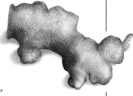

GINGER

> ***Tea:*** *Boil 1 oz of dried ginger root in 1 cup water for 15 to 20 minutes.*

TIP*385*

CUT DEEPLY INTO FAT

According to the USDA Dietary Guidelines, your total fat intake should be at or below 30 percent of your total daily calories. But many scientists think that recommendation does not go far enough; they recommend aiming for a 20 percent fat diet. Good evidence suggests that people who restrict their dietary fat even lower, to 10 percent of total calories, and who make other lifestyle changes, such as exercising regularly and practicing stress-reduction techniques, not only significantly reduce their risk of heart disease, but can actually help clear existing clogged arteries.

TIP *386*

DO A FAT SWITCH

Although you should restrict your total fat consumption, some fats are better for your heart than others. Saturated fats—the ones found mostly in meat, butter, cheese, coconut oil, palm oil, and the hydrogenated vegetable oils used in many processed foods—are the worst. They raise your blood cholesterol. On the other hand, polyunsaturated fats—primarily found in some fish and in corn, safflower and soybean oils—can actually lower your blood cholesterol. So read food labels carefully and, whenever possible, replace foods high in saturated fats with those high in polyunsaturated ones.

TIP *387*

AN OKAY TO OLIVE OIL

Recent research has shown that a third kind of dietary fat—monounsaturated fat—not only helps lower total cholesterol levels, but also specifically lowers the "bad" low-density lipo-proteins (LDLs). Olive oil is high in monounsaturated fat, as are nuts, avocados, canola oil and peanut oil.

TIP *388*

NEW NEWS ON
WEIGHTLIFTING

In the past, physicians usually warned people with high blood
pressure against lifting weights, because it can temporarily raise
blood pressure to dangerous levels. Recent research, however,
has shown that a type of weightlifting called circuit training,
which uses relatively light weights on a series of weight machines,
raises blood pressure only slightly and within safe limits. It also
provides a moderate aerobic workout, which is good for the
heart. Be sure, however, to clear any weightlifting program with
your doctor before getting started.

TIP *389*

IT'S ABOUT TIME

Research has shown that the heart appears most able to tolerate
heavy stress around 5:00 p.m., and the least able to handle it
around 9:00 a.m., which is when most heart attacks occur. So
if you are at increased risk of heart disease, you may want to
schedule your day in such a way that the more stressful activities
on your calendar occur in the afternoon.

TIP *390*

DRINK PLENTY OF WATER

If you suffer from bronchitis, emphysema, or other respiratory
illness, be sure to drink four to six 8-oz glasses of water or
other fluids daily. The fluid will thin the mucus in your inflamed upper bronchial passages. This in turn will make it
easier to cough up the mucus.

TIP *391*

AVOID DEHYDRATING LIQUIDS

Cross alcohol and caffeinated beverages such as coffee, tea, and
cola off your fluid list if you have bronchitis. These liquids are de-
hydrating and may actually cause you to lose more fluids than you
take in. The less liquid in your system, the greater the difficulty in
coughing up excess mucus.

TIP *392*

STEER CLEAR OF SMOKE

If you have any kind of respiratory illness, such as bronchitis,
asthma, or emphysema, not only should you not smoke, you
should also stay out of rooms where anyone else is smoking.
Being in a house where people smoke is especially dangerous
for children with asthma.

TIP *393*

INVEST IN A VAPORIZER

A cool-water vaporizer can help shorten a bout with bronchitis by producing moisture that will loosen the mucus inside your lungs, thus making it easier for you to cough up phlegm. A vaporizer is most effective when used in a small space, such as a bathroom, where it can create the density of steam necessary to be truly helpful. Be sure to clean the vaporizer regularly to prevent the spread of germs.

TIP *394*

THE SINK METHOD

You can also vaporize clogged bronchial and nasal passages by filling a sink full of hot water, covering your head with a towel, and breathing in the steam. To make the steam even more effective, try adding to the water a few drops of one of the following essential oils: eucalyptus *(Eucalyptus globulus),* hyssop *(Hyssopus officinalis),* aniseed *(Pimpinella anisum),* lavender *(Lavandula officinalis),* pine *(Pinus sylvestris),* or rosemary *(Rosmarinus officinalis).*

LAVENDER

TIP *395*

BRING OUT THE HANDKERCHIEF

To help ease congested bronchial or nasal passages when you can't be near a humidifier or steaming sink, carry a handkerchief or tissue dabbed with a few drops of eucalyptus *(Eucalyptus globulus)* or lavender *(Lavandula officinalis)* oil. Whenever breathing becomes difficult, hold the scented handkerchief to your nose and inhale.

TIP *396*

AN HERBAL EXPECTORANT

COLTSFOOT

The herb coltsfoot *(Tussilago farfara)* may relax constricted or spasming bronchial tubes and gently help to loosen phlegm. *Infusion: Add a cup of boiling water to 1 or 2 tsp of coltsfoot; let the infusion steep for 10 minutes. Drink it as hot as possible, three times daily.*

TIP *397*

THE HOT-PEPPER TREATMENT

Eating hot red peppers, curry, and other spicy foods not only will make your eyes and nose run, it will also help you cough up excess phlegm by thinning the mucus in your lungs and bronchial passages. So when you find yourself battling bronchitis, try adding a little more spice to your meals.

TIP *398*

BLOW UP A BALLOON

For relief from a persistent breathing problem, such as chronic bronchitis or emphysema, try blowing up balloons. One study reported that people with breathing conditions who blew into balloons 40 times a day for eight weeks showed a significant improvement in their breathing. They experienced less breathlessness and could walk farther during a six-minute period than before beginning the balloon regimen. Experts theorize that balloon blowing helps increase lung capacity.

TAKE A DEEP BREATH

You can help increase the efficiency of your lungs and strengthen the muscles that control breathing with this simple breathing exercise: While lying on your back, put the fingertips of one hand over your diaphragm, which lies immediately below your rib cage in the center of your abdomen; place your other hand on your chest. Inhale deeply through your nose and concentrate on pushing your diaphragm against your fingers; then press your chest up against your other hand. Count slowly to three, then exhale to the count of six. When you can take about a dozen breaths this way without tiring, try the exercise while sitting, then while walking, and eventually while climbing stairs.

TAKE A WALK

Physical fitness is very important for people with chronic bronchitis or emphysema, and daily walking is one of the best means to that end. Begin with a short walk and increase your distance every day. Try to avoid highly polluted areas, or do your walking indoors, perhaps at a local shopping mall.

TIP *401*

YOGA BREATHING

Here are two yoga exercises that can help you learn to breathe more efficiently:

- With your fingertips on your shoulders, breathe in, then breathe out and join your elbows together in front of you. Open your elbows, and lean as far back as you can. Repeat slowly, 10 times.
- While sitting on a stool or standing, make a breast-stroke motion with your arms; slowly stretch them behind you. Clasp your hands, lowering your arms below your buttocks, and pull your shoulders back. Then, still clasping your hands behind you, breathe in and lift your arms up as far as you can. Breathe out, and lower your arms. Repeat slowly, 10 times, then unclasp your hands.

TIP *402*

TAKE A TEA BREATHER

If you suffer from shortness of breath due to emphysema or chronic bronchitis, try drinking teas made from any of the following herbs: grindelia *(Grindelia* spp.), euphorbia *(Euphorbia pilulifera),* lobelia *(Lobelia inflata),* wild black cherry *(Prunus serotina)* bark, licorice *(Glycyrrhiza glabra),* motherwort *(Leonurus cardiaca),* and aniseed *(Pimpinella anisum).* Lobelia is effective but has some dangerous side effects if you take too much. Consult an herbalist or a qualified practitioner.

LOBELIA

TIP 403

FOR NIGHTTIME BREATHLESSNESS

If emphysema or chronic bronchitis worsens at night, try sipping mullein *(Verbascum thapsus)* tea before bedtime. Mullein is said to soothe mucous membranes, especially during episodes of nighttime breathlessness.

Tea: Steep 1 to 2 tsp of dried mullein leaves, flowers, or roots per cup of boiling water for 10 to 15 minutes.

MULLEIN

TIP 404

HOMEOPATHY FOR SPECIFIC SYMPTOMS

To help relieve breathing problems, try taking the following substances twice a day for a week, or as needed.

- *Antimonium tartaricum* (6c) for wheezing and congestion.
- *Ammonium carbonicum* (6c) for symptoms that worsen on damp days, in stuffy rooms, or early in the morning.
- *Hepar sulphuris* (6c) for symptoms that grow worse at night or in cold air and drafts.

TIP 405

WATCH WHAT YOU EAT

Some nutritionists recommend that people with chronic breathing problems avoid foods that cause excess mucus production, such as dairy products, sugar, processed foods, and any product that includes white flour as an ingredient.

TIP *406*

MASSAGE YOUR FOOT

Practitioners of reflexology recommend that people with congested lungs or bronchial passages do the following foot manipulation: Massage the skin between the big toe and second toe on both feet; this area is said to correspond to your throat and lungs. Then, flexing so the toes are spread apart, massage the ball of the foot, the area said to correspond to the lungs and chest.

TIP *407*

GET A LUNG METER

If you suffer from asthma, talk to your doctor about monitoring the shifts in your lung capacity at home with a peak flow meter, a device he or she can prescribe for you. The meter can alert you to reductions in your ability to exhale so you can take precautions and lessen the severity of an asthma episode.

TIP *408*

ACUPRESSURE FOR ASTHMA

To relieve some of the discomfort of asthma, try applying pressure to two acupressure points known as Bladder 13 *(illustration, below)* and Kidney 27. To find Kidney 27, put your fists on your chest, thumbs pointing upward and feel for the sensitive spot next to the breastbone, just under the collarbone. Press firmly for two minutes.

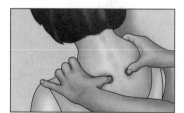

Bladder 13
Use your thumbs or fingers to press into the muscles one-half inch outward from either side of the spine and one finger width below the upper tip of the shoulder blade. Take 5 deep breaths, then release.

TIP *409*

HOMEOPATHY FOR ASTHMA

A number of homeopathic remedies are available for treating asthma symptoms, including the following:

- *Arsenicum album* (30c) to help calm restlessness and anxiety; take as required.
- *Aconite* (30c) for symptoms that worsen at night or during cold weather, or that come on very suddenly; take as required.
- *Natrum sulphuricum* (30c) for symptoms exacerbated by dampness; take as required.

TIP *410*

ROOT OUT EXCESS MUCUS

To help clear your body of excess mucus that may be inhibiting your breathing, try an infusion made from elecampane *(Inula helenium)*, a root that acts as a soothing expectorant.

Infusion: Shred the root to yield 1 tsp and add a full cup of cold water; let the infusion stand for 10 hours, then strain and drink it hot three times daily.

TIP *411*

PIGEON BREATH

If you have a breathing problem, try the yoga position known as the Pigeon.

Pigeon
From a kneeling position, slide your left leg straight behind you and place your right knee between your hands. Inhale and stretch up through your torso while arching your back slightly. Release, then repeat on the other side.

TIP *412*

VITAMINS FOR ASTHMA

A daily dose of B complex vitamins (50 to 100 mg) and magnesium (400 to 600 mg) may help reduce the frequency and severity of asthma episodes.

TIP *413*

TRACE YOUR TRIGGERS

To identify the allergens that trigger your asthma attacks, keep a detailed journal. Write down all the environmental and emotional factors that affect you every day over the course of several months. When you have an asthma attack, go back to your journal to see which factor, or combination of factors, might have contributed to it.

TIP *414*

ANCIENT ASTHMA REMEDY

For asthma, Chinese practitioners recommend an ancient cinnamon twig decoction.

Decoction: Mix 9 grams cinnamon (Cinnamomum cassia) twigs, 9 grams white peony root, 9 grams ginger (Zingiber officinale), 6 grams Chinese licorice (Glycyrrhiza uralensis), and 12 pieces Chinese dates. Steep the mixture in cold water, then bring to a boil. Drink it hot.

TIP 415

KEEP THE AIR CLEAN

If your breathing problems are related to allergies, consider installing a high-efficiency air cleaner in your home to remove pollen and mold spores, two common allergens. Also use an air conditioner in your home and car during warm seasons to keep pollen out.

TIP 416

HIRE A DUST-MITE BUSTER

Consider hiring a special cleaning service to rid your carpeting and upholstery of dust mites, microscopic insects that live in the dust that collects on carpets and furniture. An allergy to dust mites is a leading cause of asthma.

TIP 417

BARE YOUR FLOORS

If heavy-duty rug and upholstery cleaning fails to lessen your dust mite problem enough to let you breathe more easily, then you may need to take more drastic action. Remove thick carpeting, heavy drapes, and upholstered furniture from your home. Put plastic covers on mattresses and pillows. Keep floors clean. Avoid down (feathers) in comforters, clothing, sleeping bags, and pillows. And wear a mask when vacuuming.

TIP*418*

A DECONGESTANT RUB

To relieve nasal congestion, massage the following lotion into the skin around your sinuses once a day.

Lotion: *Mix 1 drop each of the oils of lavender (Lavandula angustifolia) and niaouli (Melaleuca viridiflora)with 1 tsp of a carrier oil such as sweet almond or sunflower.*

TIP*419*

A POINT FOR HAY FEVER

To relieve breathing difficulties associated with hay fever and other respiratory allergies, try applying pressure to the acupressure point known as Large Intestine 4.

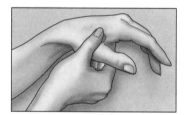

Large Intestine 4
Use the thumb and index finger of your right hand to squeeze the webbing between the thumb and index finger of your left hand. Switch hands and then repeat. (Do not apply pressure to this point if you are pregnant.)

TIP*420*

AVOID ASPIRIN

Aspirin and ibuprofen may actually worsen symptoms of hay fever and asthma. The overuse of aspirin can also cause nasal polyps to form in some susceptible people. If you have any of these conditions, use other types of pain relievers.

TIP *421*

A CAUTIONARY TALE

When using over-the-counter nose drops or spray to clear up a stuffy nose or chest, be sure to follow directions carefully. Over-use of these products can cause your mucous membranes to produce more fluid, making the congestion even worse than it was. Never use one of these products more frequently or longer than directed on the label. To avoid side effects, try homeopathic nasal sprays to clear up your congested sinuses, nose, or chest.

TIP *422*

HOMEOPATHY FOR NASAL POLYPS

To decrease some of the discomfort and problems caused by nasal polyps, homeopaths recommend the following:

- *Calcarea carbonica* (30c) if the polyps are accompanied by loss of smell, swelling around the bridge of the nose, and yellow mucus.
- *Phosphorus* (30c) if the polyps bleed easily.
- *Psorinum* (30c) or *Thuja* (30c) if mucus drips down the back of the throat and you feel weak and chilled.
- *Teucrium* (30c) if the polyps are accompanied by sneezing and a crawling sensation in the nose, and mucus forms into large dry pieces.

For the best remedy for you, check with a homeopathic physician.

TIP *423*

OILS FOR BLOCKED SINUSES

To help open up clogged sinuses, try swabbing your nasal passages with oil of bitter orange, or massage your face with essence of lavender mixed into vegetable oil.

TIP 424

WARM RELIEF

For immediate relief from the pain of blocked sinuses, place a warm, wet compress on your nose. The heat will help open your sinuses. For added effectiveness, add a drop or two of menthol or eucalyptus *(Eucalyptus globulus)* to the compress.

TIP 425

FOR SWOLLEN SINUSES

To relieve the pain, congestion, and swelling of sinusitis, apply pressure to the acupressure point known as Large Intestine 20.

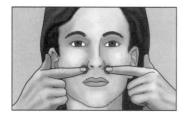

Large Intestine 20
Using your index or middle fingers, press hard on the points on the outer edge of the nostrils at the base of the nose.

TIP 426

WESTERN HERBS
FOR SINUSITIS

To help reduce the excessive mucus production associated with sinusitis, Western herbalists recommend drinking teas made from elder *(Sambucus nigra)* flower, eyebright *(Euphrasia officinalis)*, marsh mallow *(Althaea officinalis)*, or goldenrod *(Solidago virgaurea)*.

EYEBRIGHT

TIP 427

EASTERN HERBS FOR SINUSITIS

Chinese herbalists recommend the following herbs for the treatment of sinusitis symptoms: honeysuckle *(Lonicera japonica)*, fritillary bulb *(Fritillaria cirrhosa)*, tangerine peel *(Citrus reticulata)*, xanthium fruit *(Xanthium sibiricum)*, and magnolia flower *(Magnolia liliflora)*.

TIP 428

TRY ACUPUNCTURE

If your sinusitis is causing you much discomfort, you may want to seek the care of an acupuncturist. Studies have shown that acupuncture can be effective in draining blocked sinuses. Be sure to consult a licensed practitioner.

TIP 429

HOMEOPATHY FOR SINUSITIS

To relieve symptoms associated with sinusitis, homeopaths recommend the following:

- *Kali bichromicum* (30c) once or twice a day for acute sinusitis with thick, stringy mucus and pain in the cheeks or the bridge of the nose.
- *Mercurius vivus* (30c) twice a day for sinusitis with intense facial pain, alternating chills and sweat, and yellow-green discharge from the nose and mouth.
- *Nux vomica* (30c) twice a day for acute sinusitis with a clear, thin discharge, sneezing, headache, and a stuffy nose at night.
- *Pulsatilla* (30c) twice a day for sinusitis with light yellow or green nasal discharge accompanied by low spirits and lack of thirst.

Skin, Hair, Teeth, and Nails

TIP *430*

NO ROUGH STUFF

If you suffer from acne, wash your face gently with your fingertips, using an unscented, oilfree soap, calendula soap, or a specially medicated bar. Scrubbing your face with abrasives or rough cloths can actually aggravate acne by damaging already inflamed skin and spreading the infection.

TIP *431*

BEFORE ACNE STRIKES

Apply a gel or cream containing benzoyl peroxide to all areas of the face that are prone to breakouts, even when no pimples are present. Benzoyl peroxide fights mild to moderate acne in two ways: by subduing fatty acid cells that irritate the skin and by killing bacteria in facial pores. Start with a lower concentration—2.5 to 5 percent—and work up to 10 percent only if your face doesn't become excessively dry.

TIP *432*

READ THE LABEL

Adult women who suffer from more than a periodic pimple or two should check the labels of their facial cosmetics. Heavy oils in makeup are a likely culprit when it comes to acne after adolescence. Look for a water-based foundation, and also avoid lanolin, sodium lauryl sulfate, laureth-4, and isopropyl myristate, which are often too rich for sensitive facial skin.

TIP 433

TOO-ROSY CHEEKS

Abnormally flushed cheeks and nose—a condition called
rosacea—can be curtailed by reducing or eliminating spicy
foods, caffeine, alcohol, and hot drinks from your diet.
The condition also responds well to supplements of B vitamins, especially riboflavin (vitamin B_2).

TIP 434

CHOICES FOR ATHLETE'S FOOT

Soak feet infected with athlete's foot fungus in warm, salted
water (1 tsp salt per cup) for 5 to 10 minutes every day and dry
thoroughly. Then apply a baking soda paste between your toes;
an aluminum chloride solution, available from any pharmacy;
the herb tea tree oil (*Melaleuca* spp.); or an over-the-counter
product containing undecylenic acid or the antifungal drugs
clotrimazole or miconazole. Never tear off flaking skin, since
you can damage healthy skin nearby and spread the infection.

TIP 435

SOOTHING A BLISTER

If you have a blister caused by friction, soothe the skin with
calendula *(Calendula officinalis)* ointment, which also
has antiseptic properties that help keep infection at bay.
The blister acts as a natural dressing over the new skin
beneath, so avoid popping or tearing it. For fastest
healing, keep the area protected from dirt during the
day with an adhesive bandage or, for larger blisters, a
gauze pad and adhesive tape, but uncover it and expose   CALENDULA
it to air while you sleep so the skin can toughen.

173

TIP *436*

SOCKS & SHOES

If blisters are a problem for you, wear socks shaped with heels rather than tube socks, which bunch up and cause blisters, and opt for acrylic and other synthetic fibers, which generate less friction than cotton or wool. You can prevent blisters caused by stiff new shoes by putting petroleum jelly or an adhesive bandage on your heels before stepping out.

TIP *437*

TURN OFF THE SWEAT

Excessive sweating may be linked to a zinc deficiency. Taking a 30- to 60-mg supplement a day may help solve the problem.

TIP *438*

TREATING A BOIL

Warm compresses or a warm Epsom salt bath will help draw the pus out of a boil. Keep the infection, which is caused by staph bacteria, from spreading by using an over-the-counter antibacterial ointment, covering the boil with an adhesive bandage—and resisting the urge to squeeze.

TIP *439*

DON'T BUTTER THAT BURN

Immediately flush minor burns with cold running water, then apply a cold compress. Contrary to myth, butter can exacerbate a burn by holding in the heat and slowing down healing. Use calendula *(Calendula officinalis)* cream instead.

TIP *440*

THE POISON IVY ITCH

For the relief of discomfort caused by poison ivy, it's hard to beat the old standby calamine lotion, which cools the skin and absorbs oozing from the rash. Apply it three or four times a day until the oozing stops. As an alternative, mix cornstarch, oatmeal, baking soda, or Epsom salt with just enough water to make a thick paste, and apply it directly to the rash. Or try running hot water—as hot as you can stand— over the affected skin; the itching will intensify for a moment, but then it will subside completely for several hours.

POISON IVY

TIP *441*

WHEN POISON IVY
IS A TRUE EMERGENCY

There are times when exposure to urushiol—the toxic resin found in poison oak and poison sumac, as well as poison ivy—must be considered a medical emergency. If you have breathed in the smoke from any of these plants burning, urushiol—which is not inactivated by fire—can cause a severe internal allergic reaction and must be treated immediately. Also, a skin rash that appears near your eyes, covers a large portion of your body, or shows up less than 12 hours after contact with the plant rather than the usual 24 to 48, indicating extreme sensitivity, requires medical attention. Call your doctor right away.

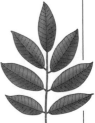

POISON OAK

POISON SUMAC

TIP 442

PAIN IN THE MOUTH

Speed healing of canker sores by rinsing four times a day with
a homemade mouthwash containing 2 oz hydrogen peroxide
and 1 tsp baking soda—both antiseptics—in a solution of 2 oz
water and 1 tsp salt. Don't swallow. If the unpleasant taste both-
ers you, try calendula *(Calendula officinalis)* tincture mixed
50/50 with water.

TIP 443

AN OUNCE OF PREVENTION

Try taking daily supplements of immunity-boosting vitamin C,
vitamin B complex, folic acid, iron, and zinc if you frequently
suffer from canker sores. Most sores show up when stress is high
and immunity is low—during adolescence and just before menstruation, in particular. Also, eat at least 4 tbsp of live-culture
yogurt every day; the bacteria it contains will help keep your system healthy.

TIP 444

THE END OF COLD SORES

Take 500-mg supplements of the amino acid lysine every day if
you develop more than three cold sores a year, and double the
dosage when you feel the tingling that indicates one is on its way.
Regardless of frequency, anyone who gets the sores should avoid
foods high in another amino acid, arginine, because the herpes
simplex virus that causes cold sores thrives on it. Such foods to
steer clear of include nuts, seeds, and chocolate.

TIP 445

CALLUS TREATMENT

Soak your feet in a warm Epsom salt bath every day to soothe and soften corns and calluses, and apply aloe *(Aloe barbadensis)*, a calendula *(Calendula officinalis)* ointment, or hydrocortisone cream if a callus becomes cracked. The best and only sure-fire remedy, though, is finding and eliminating the source of the friction or pressure that is causing the corn or callus in the first place—typically, ill-fitting shoes, and especially high heels.

TIP 446

WASH AND WEAR

Always wash new clothes, sheets, and towels before wearing or using them, to remove processing chemicals from the fabric. Until they are rinsed away, these substances can cause rashes, hives, and other skin inflammation, especially in babies and others with sensitive skin. It's also a good idea to double-rinse your clothes, and especially diapers, to remove irritating detergents.

TIP 447

BAUBLES, BANGLES, AND BEADS

When shopping for earrings, look for surgical steel or gold. The nickel used in plated jewelry frequently causes allergic rashes and cysts—which may or may not appear on your earlobe. If you develop an inexplicable rash around your mouth or painful bumps behind your ears from time to time, weed plated earrings out of your collection.

TIP *448*

COMBATTING
WINTER DRYNESS

For all-over dryness, add over-the-counter oatmeal or cornstarch preparations to a warm—but not hot—bath and soak for up to 15 minutes to allow your skin to absorb water. Pat your skin mostly dry, then immediately seal the moisture in with a generous application of lotion that is free of potentially irritating perfumes and preservatives. Rub petroleum jelly into extremely dry areas such as feet and elbows.

TIP *449*

EAT WELL FOR HEALTHY SKIN

Make sure your diet contains enough of the vitamins A, B complex, and E, as well as the mineral zinc, if your skin is frequently dry or inflamed from food allergies or reactions to metals and chemicals. These nutrients are especially beneficial for the skin, and they enhance your resistance to stress, which can cause or exacerbate flare-ups.

TIP *450*

COPING WITH ECZEMA

Soothe mild eczema with warm compresses or a bath, followed by an application of petroleum jelly or calendula (*Calendula officinalis*) ointment. Prevent babies with eczema sores from scratching—and opening up more sores—by keeping their fingernails trimmed very short and covering their hands with mittens when possible. Open eczema sores make a person extra susceptible to viral skin diseases, so keep your baby far away from anyone with cold sores or warts. Adults are wise to follow the same precaution.

TIP 451

ICING HIVES

Rub an ice cube over individual hives to keep the swelling down and numb the itch. Cold is one of the most effective ways to combat hives topically, while over-the-counter antihistamines such as diphenhydramine or chlorpheniramine work from the inside out to shrink swelling in mild cases, although they can cause drowsiness. The homeopathic remedy *Apis* (30c) might do the same job without drowsiness. Another internal remedy: An infusion of valerian *(Valeriana officinalis)*, passionflower *(Passiflora incarnata)*, or peppermint *(Mentha piperita)* may quiet stress-related hives. Sit back, relax, and sip.

VALERIAN

TIP 452

IMPETIGO INVASION

Don't use over-the-counter antibacterial ointments on the red, oozing blisters of impetigo, because these products are too weak to kill the strep and staph bacteria causing the infection. In fact, you may even spread the infection to healthy skin. Instead, mix goldenseal *(Hydrastis canadensis)* powder with calendula *(Calendula officinalis)* ointment and apply to blisters with a cotton swab. The mixture seals the wound so the infection won't spread, and the herbs help kill the bacteria.

TIP 453

FOR PLANTAR WARTS
TRY ASPIRIN

When a plantar wart sprouts on the sole of your foot, crush half an aspirin tablet, dab it on the wart, and cover with adhesive tape; leave it on for a day or two. The salicylic acid in aspirin irritates the skin, stimulating the immune system to fight the wart virus.

TIP 454

HERBS FOR THE HEAD

Use an herbal rinse instead of tar-based shampoos when you have psoriasis on your scalp.

> **Rinse.** *Pour a pint of boiling water over 1 oz each of dried rosemary (Rosmarinus officinalis) and sage (Salvia officinalis), let the mixture steep overnight, and strain. Rinse your head daily with the solution after shampooing.*

SAGE

TIP 455

PSORIASIS NO-NOS

If you suffer from psoriasis, avoid alcohol, a diet high in protein and low in fiber, and the drug ibuprofen, all of which can make the condition worse.

TIP 456

SPF ALWAYS

For maximum effectiveness, apply sunscreen with a sun protection factor of at least 15 half an hour before going outside, and again after swimming—and never let your children go out without a generous slathering. Just one bad sunburn during childhood appears to double the chance of the deadly skin cancer melanoma later in life.

TIP 457

KEEP AN EYE OUT
FOR SKIN CANCER

Report an unusual skin lesion to a doctor at once, especially if you have a family history of melanoma. Any existing mole that changes size, shape, texture, or color is especially suspect.

TIP 458

SUN SENSE

The best way to prevent sunburn is to limit your exposure to direct sunlight. The harshest rays beat down from 10:00 a.m. to 3:00 p.m., and radiation exposure is even greater at higher altitudes and southern latitudes. Also, water reflects the sun's rays and can double the dose to your skin.

TIP 459

TAKE THE SIZZLE
OUT OF SUNBURN

Over-the-counter calendula *(Calendula officinalis)* ointment or aloe *(Aloe barbadensis)* gels relieve the dryness and irritation of sunburn. Apply them liberally and often.

TIP 460

SHOCK TREATMENT
FOR VARICOSE VEINS

Hot and cold baths may slow the progress of varicose veins on the feet and ankles: Dip your feet in hot water for one to two minutes, then in cold for 30 seconds, alternating back and forth for 15 minutes.

TIP **461**

HERBS IN THE BLOOD

Take supplements of ginkgo *(Ginkgo biloba)*, hawthorn *(Crataegus laevigata)*, or bilberry *(Vaccinium myrtillus)* to strengthen blood vessels and improve circulation if you are prone to varicose veins.

HAWTHORN

TIP **462**

WART WARS

You may be able to vanquish warts by rubbing or dotting any of the following on them:

- vitamin A or E.
- a thick paste of crushed vitamin C tablets and water.
- a paste of crushed aspirin.
- aloe *(Aloe barbadensis)* or dandelion *(Taraxacum officinale)* juices.
- Thuja ointment, a classic herbal treatment for warts.

TIP **463**

DEALING WITH DANDRUFF

Massage tea tree oil *(Melaleuca* spp.) into your scalp to prevent flaking and protect against infection. The massaging action will also improve the circulation in the skin and help keep it from drying and cracking.

TEA TREE

TIP *464*

HELP FOR DRY HAIR

Your kitchen may contain the secret to lustrous tresses. After shampooing, condition your hair with plain mayonnaise or a combination of overripe banana and avocado; leave the conditioner on for five minutes to an hour, then rinse thoroughly with warm water.

TIP *465*

AN ASTRINGENT FOR OILY HEADS

For very oily hair, mix a 1-to-1 solution of witch hazel and antiseptic mouthwash, and apply it with cotton balls to the scalp after shampooing, avoiding the hair. The combination helps reduce oil production in the glands of the scalp.

TIP *466*

BRUSH THE NATURAL WAY

Keep your hair looking healthy by brushing with a moderately stiff, natural-bristle brush, which will not tear your locks. Begin with 10 to 20 strokes a day and work up to 100, using full but gentle strokes and brushing from the scalp to the tips to distribute the hair's protective natural oils. Avoid brushing hair when it is wet and especially fragile.

TIP 467

TOOTHACHE FIRST AID

A sudden toothache may be caused by food impacted between two teeth. Floss gently to remove the offending food particles and you should feel instant relief. If flossing doesn't help, your pain may be caused by infection or an impacted tooth, both of which require a dentist's attention.

TIP 468

HYPERSENSITIVE IN THE TOOTH

Use a toothpaste made for sensitive teeth and a soft-bristled brush if your teeth react to hot and cold. Such hypersensitivity can be brought on by age, receding gums, dental surgery, or excessive brushing with whitening toothpastes or hard-bristle brushes.

TIP 469

THOSE PEARLY WHITES

You can help remove stains on your teeth by brushing gently with a homemade paste of baking soda and a few drops of hydrogen peroxide. Don't use so-called whitening tooth polishes, which take off your enamel along with the stains, eventually exposing the darker layer beneath and ushering in a host of other problems in the bargain.

TIP *470*

INGROWN TOENAILS

For stubborn cases, soak your foot in warm water containing
salt or calendula *(Calendula officinalis)* (1 tbsp tincture per
pint of water), then apply an over-the-counter topical solution
formulated for ingrown nails. Once you can lift the nail away
from the skin, put a thin strand of cotton under the corner, and
change the cotton daily until the nail grows out. Prevent recurrences by wearing shoes that fit properly and clipping your nails
straight across.

TIP *471*

NAILS AU NATUREL

Remove old nail polish with acetate-based rather than acetone
solutions; they are less irritating. If your nails are brittle or split
easily, you may be allergic to polishes or adhesives for false nails;
try going without them for six months while your nails grow
out to see if the problem clears up.

TIP *472*

SPOTS BEFORE YOUR EYES

If you see white spots in your fingernails, take a multivitamin and
mineral supplement; most likely you have a zinc or vitamin B_6 deficiency. Beware of spots that come in other colors, though, such
as greenish black or bluish gray. These indicate more serious
problems, including infection or heart disease, and they require
medical attention.

TIP 473

BURPLESS STRATEGIES

Eat at a slow, relaxed pace—as opposed to wolfing down your food—to reduce the amount of air you swallow during ingestion. Less air in means less air out. Three things to avoid if you prefer not to burp: drinking with a straw, carbonated beverages, and chewing gum.

TIP 474

IT MIGHT BE MILK

Sometimes, gas pains result from lactose intolerance, an inability to digest the primary sugar found in milk. If milk and milk products give you problems, try supplements of the digestive enzyme lactase, which can help you break down milk sugars. If this doesn't help, consider substituting soy milk for cow's milk.

TIP 475

DIETARY NO-NOS

Besides limiting your intake of beans and peas, you can reduce gas production by avoiding fermented foods such as cheese, soy sauce, and alcohol. It also helps if you don't consume proteins and carbohydrates at the same meal.

TIP*476*

OVER-THE-COUNTER HELP

If you're suffering from garden-variety gas pains, try nonprescription products containing the ingredient simethicone, which serves to break up gas bubbles in the large intestine. Or chew on 8 to 10 fennel seeds after you are finished eating.

TIP*477*

LIQUID RELIEF

To minimize the discomfort of intestinal gas, make anise water by steeping 1 tsp of aniseeds *(Pimpinella anisum)* in a cup of water for 10 minutes. Herbal teas can also help, especially those made from peppermint *(Mentha piperita),* chamomile *(Matricaria recutita),* or fennel *(Foeniculum vulgare).*

PEPPERMINT

TIP*478*

CREATING A GAS SHORTAGE

To reduce the amount of intestinal gas that often results from eating beans, try an over-the-counter product containing alpha-galactosidase. Follow label directions.

TIP**479**

BENEFICIAL SPICE

Season beans with asafetida powder. This spice is not only flavorful, it also helps to dispel intestinal gas.

TIP**480**

FRENCH CLAY CURE

To absorb impurities and gas in your intestinal tract, dissolve two tsp of superfine white, green, or yellow French clay in a glass of water and drink at least once daily between meals. You can find French clay at health food stores.

TIP**481**

DEPRESSURE GAS
WITH ACUPRESSURE

For gas pain relief, try pressing acupressure points known as Conception Vessel 6 and Stomach 36.

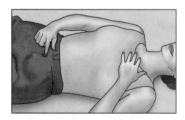

Conception Vessel 6
Measure three finger widths below the navel, then press inward on this point as far as you can, using your index finger. Inhale slowly and deeply, relaxing as you exhale.

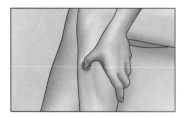

Stomach 36
Measure four finger widths below the kneecap just outside the shinbone (flex your foot; you should feel a muscle bulge at the point site). Press the point steadily with a finger or thumb, then repeat on the other leg.

TIP *482*

WHEN TO CALL THE DOCTOR

Call your doctor if you have persistent bloating for more than three days, or if your flatulence is accompanied by severe abdominal pains, weight loss, or any other unusual symptoms. In most cases, however, realize that it's normal to pass gas 10 times or more per day.

TIP *483*

DIGESTIVE FOOTPRINT

Try reflexology to keep your digestive system operating smoothly. Manually work the following areas of your feet to improve organ functioning—the stomach areas to encourage digestion, liver to trigger bile secretion, gall bladder to release stored bile, intestine to stimulate regular contractions, and pancreas to increase digestive enzymes.

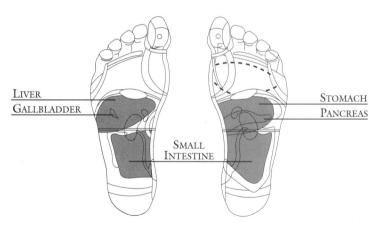

LIVER
GALLBLADDER

STOMACH
PANCREAS

SMALL
INTESTINE

TIP*484*

NASTY NITRITES

Slash your risk of stomach cancer by cutting out smoked, pickled, salted, and barbecued foods. These all contain nitrites or other nitrogen-containing compounds that are known carcinogens.

TIP*485*

ANTICANCER FOODS

To help your body protect itself from stomach cancer, drink herb tea, eat garlic, and consume plenty of fresh fruits and vegetables each day.

TIP*486*

WARNING SIGNS

Consult with your healthcare practitioner if abdominal discomfort lasts longer than a few weeks, or if you have unusually dark stools, a possible indication of intestinal bleeding. The most likely cause is a stomach ulcer, although your doctor will want to rule out other possibilities.

TIP*487*

HEARTBURN:
AVOID THE USUAL SUSPECTS

If you suffer frequent acid indigestion and heartburn, avoid smoking, caffeine, decaffeinated beverages, alcohol, gulping your food, and nonsteroidal anti-inflammatory drugs like aspirin and ibuprofen.

TIP 488

GASTROENTERITIS:
WHEN TO SEE YOUR DOCTOR

You can usually self-treat gastroenteritis, an inflammation of your digestive system, by resting and drinking lots of fluids. Symptoms include abdominal cramping or pain, nausea, diarrhea, vomiting, fever, malaise, weakness, and gas. Most of the time, these abate after a day or two. If your symptoms are severe or persistent, see your doctor or your local homeopath, who may suggest *Phosphorus, Nux vomica,* or *Arsenicum*—homeopathic remedies that may help speed the healing.

TIP 489

CLEAR LIQUIDS

If you're suffering from flu, traveler's diarrhea, or food poisoning, soothe your inflamed stomach lining or intestinal tract by drinking water or a prepared electrolyte solution available at your local pharmacy.

TIP 490

EASE THE SOLIDS

Gastritis sufferers: Consume only liquids on the first day you have symptoms, then reintroduce small quantities of bland, solid foods as tolerated on subsequent days. Many physicians recommend the BRAT diet—bananas, rice, applesauce, and toast.

TIP 491

TREAT THE CAUSE

If you experience the upper abdominal pain and other symptoms of a peptic ulcer, get tested for *Helicobacter pylori* bacteria. Doctors used to think ulcers were caused by stress and poor dietary habits, but now they know a bacterial infection of the stomach lining is often the real culprit. In many cases, antibiotic treatment can cure the condition permanently. Until antibiotics have a chance to work at the root cause of your ulcer, you can reduce the pain by resting, eating smaller, more frequent meals, taking an antacid or other medication, and avoiding cigarettes, alcohol, caffeine, and anti-inflammatory drugs

---

TIP 492

ALLEVIATE WITH LICORICE

Prepare an infusion of licorice *(Glycyrrhiza glabra)* to stimulate ulcer-healing mucus secretions by your stomach.

Infusion: Add 1 tsp shredded licorice root to a cup of water, simmer for 15 minutes, and drink hot, three times a day for no more than a few days at a time.

TIP 493

BOOST MUCIN

Try boosting your intake of zinc along with vitamins A and E to stimulate your body's production of mucin, a substance that protects the stomach lining. Another option: Drink a quart of cabbage juice each day. This contains glutamine, which some nutritionists believe stimulates mucin-producing cells. Aloe vera juice will soothe an ulcer and heal the stomach lining; drink two cups a day.

ALOE

TIP *494*

CALMING AN IRRITABLE BOWEL

If you suffer from the "out of control" digestive difficulty known as irritable bowel syndrome, try treating the condition with a combination of fiber, fluids, exercise, and stress management. Cutting back on fat and using a bulk-forming soluble fiber product like psyllium *(Plantago psyllium)* can also bring relief.

TIP *495*

DIETARY DOS AND DON'TS

If you've been diagnosed with a chronic disorder of the intestines such as ulcerative colitis or Crohn's disease, take special care to avoid spicy and high-fat foods, which can worsen diarrheal symptoms. Instead, try drinking juice made from leafy green vegetables like cabbage, or broth made from kelp. Both contain high levels of chlorophyll, which can effectively relieve symptoms in many patients.

KELP

TIP *496*

STRIKE A COBRA POSE

Try the yoga position called the Cobra to revitalize your stomach and bowels.

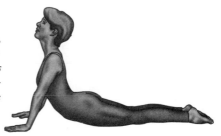

Cobra
Place both forearms on the floor, elbows directly under your shoulders. Slowly straighten your arms and arch your back until your abdomen is off the ground. Relax and slowly uncurl, lowering your torso back to the floor.

TIP*497*

SAFE HANDLING

You can prevent food poisoning by practicing good kitchen hygiene. Always refrigerate meat, seafood, and dairy products. Be sure to wash raw vegetables and fruit thoroughly. Keep a clean kitchen, and always wash your hands with soap before and after handling food.

TIP*498*

GALLSTONES

See your doctor about removing gallstones by surgery or a new, noninvasive method that pulverizes them into smaller particles. Suspect gallstones if you suffer an extreme, sudden pain in your upper-right abdomen following a fatty meal. To prevent recurrence, restrict your intake of meat and fat.

TIP*499*

A CLOVE A DAY KEEPS CRAMPING AWAY

Eat a clove of raw garlic *(Allium sativum)* daily to minimize the cramping associated with colitis.

GARLIC

TIP 500

COFFEE AND FIBER

When afflicted with diarrhea, cut back on coffee and excessive fiber intake. Within 48 hours, the diarrhea should cease.

TIP 501

DRUG-INDUCED DIARRHEA

If you develop diarrhea after beginning a new medication, tell your doctor. Antibiotics, antacids, cimetidine, quinine, and other drugs can all cause diarrhea. Your doctor may be able to adjust the dose, or switch you to another medication without this side effect.

TIP 502

ABDOMINAL RELAXATION

Try aromatherapy as a palliative for the intestinal inflammation known as diverticulitis. Inhaling 2 drops of hyssop *(Hyssopus officinalis)* three times a day can often help relax the digestive tract.

TIP *503*

HERBAL ADJUNCT

Ask your doctor about supplementing conventional treatment for mild diverticulitis—bed rest, stool softeners, liquid diet, and antibiotics—with a remedy herbalists recommend: slippery elm (*Ulmus fulva*).

Tea: *Place 1 tsp powder into ½ cup water, boil and simmer 15 minutes, and drink three times a day.*

TIP *504*

KNOW YOUR LEFT FROM RIGHT

Remember this rule of thumb for severe abdominal pain: For pain on your lower-left side, suspect diverticulitis; for pain on the right, suspect appendicitis. Either way, see your doctor.

TIP *505*

FAST UNDER ATTACK

Try a one day juice "fast" for an acute episode of diverticulitis. Slowly phase in low-bulk foods like potatoes, eventually adding cooked vegetables, fruits, and applesauce if your system tolerates them. Remember, however, to avoid all milk and milk products, from yogurt to cheese.

TIP *506*

NATURAL LAXATIVES

Avoid suppositories for constipation, because your system can easily become dependent on chemical stimulation. Instead, choose natural bulk laxatives like prunes, psyllium *(Plantago psyllium)*, or powdered flaxseed *(Linum usitatissimum)*. Taking 1 to 2 rounded tsp of psyllium a day in cold water or juice not only will keep you regular but may also enhance your cholesterol profile.

TIP *507*

EXERCISE WORKS

Exercising for 20 to 30 minutes daily, and at an intensity level sufficient to get your heart pumping strongly, is one of the best remedies for chronic constipation. Regular exercise can also help speed intestinal gas through your system.

TIP *508*

CULPRITS IN THE MEDICINE CABINET

Beware of drugs that can cause constipation. Common culprits include aluminum salts in antacids; iron and calcium supplements; morphine and codeine; and many other medications, such as antihistamines, diuretics, antidepressants, antipsychotics, and blood pressure pills. Ask your doctor's advice if you suffer this side effect.

TIP *509*

DEPENDABLE FOLK REMEDY

Try greeting each day with a glass of warm water mixed with lemon juice. This time-tested folk remedy really works to establish regularity in many people.

TIP *510*

RUBBING RELIEF
AND SOOTHING TEA

You can help reduce the discomfort of a diverticulitis attack by massaging your lower abdomen with a light vegetable oil. Use circular, clockwise strokes while lying down, then follow the massage with a cup of chamomile tea *(Matricaria recutita)* to further promote intestinal relaxation.

CHAMOMILE

TIP *511*

THE MYTH ABOUT NUTS

If you suffer from diverticulitis, don't feel you must avoid nuts and seeds in your diet; just make sure to chew them well. Despite conventional wisdom about shunning such foods, researchers have found that nuts are no more likely than any other food to become caught in diverticula.

―――――――――――● TIP *512* ●―――――――――――

REGULAR HABIT

To promote regularity, get in the habit of sitting on the toilet for 10 minutes at the same time each day (usually after a meal), regardless of whether you feel the urge to go. Be patient: Your body will eventually lock onto a regular routine, but it may take several months for this to happen. (**Caution:** If you have a tendency to develop hemorrhoids or varicose veins, this is probably not the right strategy for you; consult your doctor.) To avoid becoming constipated, never ignore the call of nature.

―――――――――――● TIP *513* ●―――――――――――

GLUTEN ALLERGY

If you suffer the lower gastrointestinal distress of celiac disease, see your doctor about eliminating all sources of gluten from your diet. Avoiding this protein, which is present in most cereal grains, can bring great relief in a matter of days, although a complete cure may take months. Ask your doctor about vitamin supplements as well.

TIP 514

LIFESTYLE CHOICES

To prevent or forestall kidney problems, practice the same healthy lifestyle choices that ward off high blood pressure, atherosclerosis, and diabetes: good diet, regular exercise, and stress management.

TIP 515

WHEN IN DOUBT, THROW IT OUT

Toss out any nuts, seeds, or rice that have become moldy from humidity. The mold could be aflatoxins, which have been linked to kidney cancer and other health problems.

TIP 516

NIX OXALIC

Never use skin bleaches or freckle removers containing oxalic acid. This kidney-damaging compound is also present in rhubarb leaves as well as some heavy-duty household cleaning and polishing products.

TIP 517

SUGAR SOLUTION

If you're diabetic, make sure to follow your doctor's recommendations for keeping your blood glucose levels within a tight range. Evidence suggests tight control of blood sugar can reduce further injury to kidneys.

TIP 518

SHUN MUSHROOMS

Never eat wild mushrooms. Even experts can have trouble distinguishing edible from poisonous varieties If you guess wrong, you can cause acute kidney disease or worse.

TIP 519

DRINK ON THE RUN

When participating in a marathon or other endurance event, make sure to drink often during the race. Dehydration hastens the breakdown of muscle tissues, which can release chemicals that severely damage kidneys.

TIP 520

DE-PRESSURIZING KIDNEYS

If you suffer from high blood pressure, ask your doctor about prescribing angiotensin-converting enzyme (ACE) inhibitors or diuretics to prevent additional damage to your kidneys.

TIP 521

BONE INSURANCE

To keep your bones from weakening due to kidney disease, take 1,500 mg of calcium each day and exercise 20 to 30 minutes, four times a week.

TIP 522

FOODS TO AVOID

For the best protection for your kidneys, don't eat organ meats like liver or kidney. Also avoid flounder, mussels, scallops, oysters, and vegetables grown.in sewage sludge fertilizers. All these foods concentrate levels of kidney-toxic metals like cadmium.

TIP 523

HERBAL WARNING

If you've been diagnosed with kidney cancer, check with your doctor before taking any medicinal herb. No herbal remedy has been shown to cure cancer—and some can actually damage kidneys further.

TIP 524

DRY-CLEANING SAFETY

Keep your car windows open when driving home from the dry cleaners to avoid inhaling a common dry-cleaning chemical, tetrachloroethylene, which is toxic to kidneys. Let dry-cleaned clothes "air out" for six hours before bringing them inside—dry-cleaned sleeping bags require several days of airing out.

TIP 525

GIVE IT A REST

If you've had urinary tract problems, avoid alcohol, coffee, salt, black tea, chocolate, carbonated drinks, citrus fruits, tomatoes, spicy foods, vinegar, artificial sweeteners, and sugar. All of these can irritate the urinary tract and add further stress to kidneys.

TIP 526

BATHROOM HYGIENE

Practice good hygiene to prevent *E. coli* bacteria from entering your urethra and spreading to your kidneys. Women should always wipe from front to back.

TIP 527

DON'T HOLD IT

Remember to void your bladder frequently—that is, whenever you feel the urge to go.

TIP 528

COOL FASHION

Create an environment inhospitable to microbes by wearing cotton underwear and loose clothes. Such garments will keep your crotch cool and wick away the humidity that provides an ideal environment for bacterial growth.

TIP *529*

CRANBERRY CURE

Drink 12 to 16 fluid oz of nonsweetened cranberry juice a day or take cranberry capsules to fight off urinary tract infections. High levels of hippuric acid in these berries hamper the growth of *E. coli* bacteria.

TIP *530*

AFTER SEX

Women should empty their bladders after intercourse to flush out any bacteria that may have been pushed inside.

TIP *531*

HERBAL CLEANSER

Women with a history of bladder infections can reduce the odds of reinfection after sex with a medicinal solution of the herb goldenseal *(Hydrastis canadensis)*.

> **Solution:** *Bring 2 tsp of dried goldenseal root per cup of water to a boil, then simmer 15 minutes. Once the solution has cooled to room temperature, use it to wash the perineal area before and after sex.*

GOLDENSEAL

TIP 532

A GOOD FIT

To help prevent infections, if you use a diaphragm, make sure it fits properly, and avoid leaving it in longer than you need to.

TIP 533

NO SCENTS

Stay away from scented soaps, bubble baths, and vaginal deodorants, all of which can irritate your urinary tract and predispose you to urinary and bladder infections.

TIP 534

WATER AND STONES

When enduring the pain of kidney stones, ask your doctor if he or she recommends that you drink six to eight glasses of water a day, even more during hot weather. Some practitioners feel this stresses the kidneys, but it might help in your case. You can also help manage the pain with aspirin or acetaminophen. Upward of 90 percent of these deposits of calcium, uric acid, or other crystals will pass from the body on their own in three to six weeks.

TIP 535

WARM COMFORT

To palliate the pain of kidney stones, place a hot-water bottle over the painful area. Cover the hot-water bottle with a towel to prevent your skin from burning.

TIP 536

STRAINING ANALYSIS

Urinate through a strainer to "catch" voided kidney stones for chemical analysis. Depending on what your stones are made of, your doctor can prescribe drugs and recommend dietary changes to prevent a future episode.

TIP 537

URIC ACID STONES

Avoid any foods that can raise uric acid levels, a common component of kidney stones. Some of the worst offenders include anchovies, sardines, organ meats, and brewer's yeast.

TIP 538

CALCIUM OXALATE STONES

Since many kidney stones are made up of calcium oxalate, be sure to avoid foods that contain calcium oxalate—including chocolate, celery, grapes, bell peppers, beans, strawberries, spinach, asparagus, and beets—and to stay away from substances that can draw calcium into the urine—such as chocolate, coffee, tea, cola, and decaffeinated beverages.

TIP *539*

SUPPLEMENTARY HELP

Take 10 mg of vitamin B$_6$ and 300 mg of magnesium daily. These supplements will reduce your body's formation of oxalates.

TIP *540*

MEDICAL PRESCRIPTION

If your kidney stones do consist of calcium oxalate, ask your doctor about ways to decrease stone formation, including prescribing a thiazide diuretic.

TIP *541*

UNBLOCKING STRATEGIES

If a kidney stone causes an infection or blocks your ureter, see your doctor immediately. Effective removal options include surgery and a new, noninvasive technique using high-energy shock waves to pulverize stones into smaller pieces that your body will be able to pass.

TIP *542*

STELLAR FRUIT

To manage pain and facilitate urination during a kidney stone episode, try eating star fruit (*Averrhoa carambola*).

Snack: *Place three fresh star fruit in a pan with 2 tsp of honey, boil until soft, then eat the fruit and its juice. Repeat every day until the stone passes and you're pain free.*

TIP 543

HELP FOR INCONTINENCE

If you suffer urinary leakage, dripping, or other symptoms of incontinence, see your doctor about the latest treatments, including medication, counseling, and surgery.

TIP 544

BAD SIGNS

Consult your health practitioner if you have cloudy, foul-smelling urine. These symptoms are frequently caused by a bacterial infection, cystitis, which can be cured with antibiotic, herbal, or homeopathic treatment.

TIP 545

EXCESSIVE URINATION

If you are urinating 3 quarts or more a day, see your doctor to rule out a variety of conditions, including—though not limited to—diabetes.

TIP 546

PAINFUL URINATION

If it hurts to urinate, with or without an accompanying discharge from the penis or vagina, seek immediate treatment. Such symptoms may mean you have contracted a sexually transmitted disease (STD), pelvic inflammatory disease (PID), or other serious infection that can put you and your sexual partner at risk.

TIP 547

COOL THE BURN

To relieve the burning sensation that accompanies a bladder infection, try mixing 1 tsp dried, crushed nettle *(Urtica dioica)*
leaves or root in a cup of boiling water. After it has cooled, take
1 tbsp every two hours, up to 1 cup a day, for anti-inflammatory
relief. Or try the homeopathic remedy *Cantharis* (30c) three
times a day.

TIP 548

TRY BEARBERRY

Try a time-tested folk remedy for bladder infections: a tea prepared
from the evergreen shrub uva ursi *(Arctostaphylos uva-ursi)*.
This herb functions both as an anti-inflammatory medicine and as a diuretic. If you don't have the time to
prepare the tea, take 3 uva ursi capsules each day until
the infection clears.

> ***Tea:*** *Soak fresh leaves of uva ursi in brandy for*
> *several hours, then add 1 tsp of these leaves to a*
> *cup of boiling water.*

UVA URSI

TIP 549

VITAMINS FOR
BLADDER RELIEF

To speed recovery from a bladder infection, take 25,000 IU of
beta carotene daily. Some patients find that 500 mg of vitamin C
taken every four or five hours can also help, but check with your
doctor first if you're also taking an antibiotic. In some cases, vitamin C can hamper the antibiotic's effectiveness.

Coping with Serious Conditions

THINGS YOU

CAN DO—AND THINGS

YOU SHOULD

KNOW—TO HELP

MANAGE AND TREAT

SERIOUS

HEALTH PROBLEMS

Coping with Serious Conditions

TIP 550

NUTRITION FOR HEAVY DRINKERS

Poor nutrition goes with heavy drinking. To aid withdrawal and recovery, alcoholics often need to restore deficient nutrients, such as vitamins A, B complex—particularly thiamine (vitamin B_1)—and C; carnitine, magnesium, selenium, and zinc; and essential fatty acids and antioxidants. One study found that recovery programs incorporating nutritional therapy were twice as effective.

Asthma
TIP 551

AN ASTHMA-BUSTING DIET

Asthmatics should avoid foods and drinks that have high concentrations of sulfites, such as beer, wine, wine vinegar, instant tea, grape juice, lemon juice, grapes, fresh shrimp, pizza dough, dried fruits (such as apricots and apples), canned vegetables, instant potatoes, corn syrup, fruit topping, and molasses. Sulfites are chemicals sometimes added to foods as a preservative, and studies have shown that they can aggravate asthma.

Bladder Cancer
TIP 552

VITAMINS AND THE BLADDER

Several scientific studies suggest that certain vitamins and minerals are beneficial in both treatment and prevention of bladder cancer. Patients receiving BCG immunotherapy may have better results with megadoses of vitamins A, B_6, C, and E, as well as zinc. Research also suggests reduced incidence of bladder cancer among people with adequate vitamin B_6, beta carotene, and selenium in their diets.

Blood Clots **TIP *553***

FISH OIL FOR STICKY BLOOD

If you want to condition your blood naturally, some authorities recommend eating more fish, believing that some fish oils make blood platelets less sticky. Certain vitamins and minerals may also act as natural anticoagulants. Ask your doctor or licensed nutrition therapist about supplemental vitamin E, magnesium, or garlic to prevent abnormal clots from forming.

Breast Cancer **TIP *554***

LUMP OR TUMOR?

In addition to having an annual medical checkup, all women should conduct monthly breast self-examinations. Several tests can help distinguish a benign lump from a malignant tumor. Feeling the lump may provide clues: A benign cyst may feel like a round, slippery bean, whereas a tumor may feel thicker and may cause dimpling of the skin above it.

Breast Cancer **TIP *555***

EXERCISE AND BREAST CANCER

Regular aerobic exercise may offer some protection against a woman's developing breast cancer. Studies have found that women who exercised vigorously and often were at least half as likely as nonexercisers to get breast cancer. Exercise can also help breast cancer patients better tolerate the side effects of radiation or chemotherapy.

TIP 556

HOMEOPATHY AND BRONCHITIS

For acute and chronic bronchitis, you might try some homeopathic remedies. Take the following three times a day, for up to
four days:

- *Aconite* (12x) to treat fever, cough, and tightness in
  the chest accompanied by anxiety.
- *Kali bichromicum* (12x) for loose white phlegm,
  cough, and irritability.
- *Phosphorus* (12x) for loss of voice, cough, thirst, sore
  throat, and exhaustion.

Consult a homeopath for the remedy that's best for you.

TIP 557

THE SEVEN WARNING SIGNS

To remember the seven early warning signs of cancer (as desig-
nated by the American Cancer Society), remember the word
CAUTION.

Change in bowel or bladder habits
A sore that does not heal
Unusual bleeding or discharge
Thickening or lump in the breast or elsewhere
Indigestion or difficulty swallowing
Obvious change in a wart or mole
Nagging cough or hoarseness

Cancer **TIP 558**

RELIEVING SIDE EFFECTS
OF CANCER TREATMENTS

- After radiation therapy, be gentle to your skin. Do not scrub it, expose it to sunlight, or wear tight clothing. Calendula *(Calendula officinalis)* ointment or aloe vera ointment is gentle and soothing, and you can ask your radiation oncologist about other nonirritating lotions.
- Eat light snacks throughout the day rather than three heavy meals. Also try eating food cold or at room temperature to avoid nausea.
- If your treatment involves lowering your white blood cell count, steer clear of sick people; tell your doctor about any fever or unusual symptoms.
- In addition to taking prescribed pain medication, try relaxation techniques such as yoga, meditation, or massage given by a friend or spouse. Acupuncture has also proved to relieve pain associated with many major illnesses. Although its effectiveness in treating cancer pain is not fully documented, it is a safe therapy that many cancer patients find beneficial.
- Some homeopathic remedies can alleviate the side effects of radiation and chemotherapy. *Silica* (6x) can help reduce hair loss. *Nux vomica* (12x) and *Phosphorus* (12x) may be particularly helpful in alleviating nausea. Consult a professional homeopath for the remedies appropriate for you.

Cirrhosis **TIP 559**

WATCH OUT FOR SHELLFISH

Cirrhosis patients should abstain from eating uncooked shellfish, which are sometimes harvested in polluted estuaries and may carry organisms that cause hepatitis or other diseases.

Eczema **TIP 560**

STRESS AND YOUR SKIN

A Swedish study of adult eczema patients found that those who used relaxation techniques along with their regular regimen of topical preparations improved much faster than those who received topical medication alone.

Food Poisoning **TIP 561**

EAT GOOD BACTERIA

To restore essential bacteria to your digestive tract after food poisoning, eat plain yogurt with active *Lactobacillus acidophilus* cultures, or take *Lactobacillus acidophilus* capsules. Avoid unfermented milk products, which may be difficult to digest.

Graves' Disease **TIP 562**

RELIEVING INFLAMED EYES

If your eyes become swollen and inflamed due to Graves' disease, here are a few at-home remedies:

- If your lids cannot close completely over your eyes, use eye patches at night. This will help keep your corneas from drying out.
- Use over-the-counter or prescription artificial tears to moisten your eyes whenever they feel dry.
- Try homeopathic eyedrops, not only for relief but also for treatment.
- If your eyes are red and swollen in the morning, sleep with your head elevated.
- Wear tinted glasses to protect your eyes from bright light, sunlight, and wind.

Heart Arrhythmias **TIP 563**

A COLD SPLASH IN THE FACE

Have you ever wondered how sea lions survive the shock of diving into frozen waters? Like other mammals, they are protected by an autonomic nervous response that immediately slows the heart rate. Humans also have this nervous response, which may be particularly significant to you if you suffer occasional bouts of tachycardia (too fast a heartbeat). Next time an attack occurs, try plunging your face into a basin of cold water. Your heart rate will temporarily plummet, which may serve to break the tachycardia.

Heart Disease **TIP 564**

VITAMINS FOR A HEALTHY HEART

Most people now know that eating foods low in cholesterol, saturated fat, and salt will help keep blood pressure low and decrease the formation of fatty deposits in blood vessels. Less known to the general public are those specific vitamins, minerals, and nutrients, such as magnesium, potassium, niacin (vitamin B_3), many other vitamin B complex supplenents, vitamin E, coenzyme Q10, L-carnitine (an amino acid), and the fatty acids in fish oils, that specifically protect against heart and arterial disease.

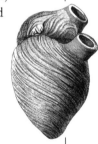

Hernia **TIP 565**

HERNIA EXERCISES

Gentle exercise on a regular basis tones and strengthens stomach muscles—and helps relieve the discomfort of a hernia. One good choice to do daily: Lie on your back with knees bent and feet on the floor. Keeping your shoulders on the floor, lift your buttocks and your lower back; gently lower yourself. Repeat 10 times.

Irritable Bowel Syndrome　　　**TIP 566**

ABDOMINAL MASSAGE

To ease bowel spasms caused by irritable bowel syndrome, try abdominal massage.

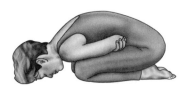

Abdominal Massage

Kneel upright and fold your arms, placing your left fist on the right side of your belly and your right hand over your left elbow. Bend at the hips and lower your forehead toward the floor. Raise your torso slowly, then switch arm positions and repeat.

Liver Cancer　　　**TIP 567**

CLEAN OUT YOUR CUPBOARD

Research shows a clear link between aflatoxins in the food supply and the incidence of primary liver cancer. Food grown in some parts of tropical Africa harbors aflatoxins, a potent carcinogen produced by a fungus in the soil. But aflatoxins are not unique to Africa—they may be lurking in the peanut butter that has been on your shelf for the past five years. Aflatoxins develop naturally in many foods—seeds, grains, rice, and nuts—as they age, especially under humid conditions. To avoid contamination, keep dry food in airtight containers and store in a cool place. Discard any food that becomes moldy, soft, rancid, or shriveled, or whose package expiration date has passed.

Lupus

TIP *568*

FOOD ALLERGIES AND LUPUS

People with lupus often have food allergies that can make symptoms worse. Identifying and avoiding problem foods can help. A change in diet may reduce inflammation and decrease pain. Nutritionists may recommend cutting down on red meat and dairy products, and increasing consumption of fish high in omega-3 fatty acids—such as mackerel, sardines, and salmon—which have anti-inflammatory properties. Alfalfa contains a substance that has been shown in tests to aggravate symptoms, so avoiding alfalfa sprouts is strongly recommended.

Macular Degeneration

TIP *569*

EATING FOR HEALTHY EYES

For macular degeneration, try a diet that includes fruits and vegetables rich in vitamin C, such as citrus fruits, cauliflower, and broccoli. Snack on nuts and seeds, which contain vitamin E. Yellow vegetables containing carotene, as well as cherries, blackberries, and blueberries, all of which contain antioxidant flavonoids, are also said to help stave off degeneration of the macula.

Manic Depression

TIP *570*

EEG BIOFEEDBACK

If you are manic depressive, try EEG biofeedback to control some of the brain-wave states underlying hyperactivity, racing thoughts, irritability, lack of sleep, and poor self-control. This therapy also seems to work for brain-wave activity associated with lower energy, low self-esteem, and poor motor coordination.

TIP 571

COPING WITH MONO

To help with the anxiety and depression that sometimes accompany long-term bouts with mono, try St.-John's-wort *(Hypericum perforatum)* or vervain *(Verbena officinalis)*. Both herbs, when taken internally, appear to act as mild sedatives. Vervain is also recommended for jaundice, one of the symptoms of mono. Make a tea out of either herb and drink three times daily. Or take in tincture form: 1 to 4 ml of St.-John's-wort or 2 to 4 ml of vervain three times a day.

ST.-JOHN'S-WORT

TIP 572

THE SWANK DIET

The best known diet for MS sufferers is the Swank Diet, devised by Dr. Roy Swank of the Oregon Health Sciences University. In many cases, it has apparently slowed the course of the disease and reduced attacks. Very low in saturated fats, it calls for specific amounts of polyunsaturated oils—sunflower and sesame oils, for example. The diet also includes proteins, supplements of cod-liver oil, and high doses of vitamins. Butter, margarine, shortening, and hydrogenated oils (such as coconut and palm) are strictly forbidden. In the first year, you are advised to avoid red meat entirely, as well as other foods high in saturated fats.

TIP 573

SWEET SUBSTITUTES

For overeaters, 1 to 2 tsp a day of brewer's yeast or some dandelion *(Taraxacum officinale)* will reduce a craving for sweets. Bee pollen or a dash of cayenne *(Capsicum annuum* var. *annuum)* may increase your metabolism.

DANDELION

TIP 574

MASSAGE AND PHLEBITIS DON'T MIX

It's quite natural to rub an aching muscle to relieve pain, but be careful if you have phlebitis. Though the risk is slight, massage—particularly vigorous massage—might dislodge a blood clot, which could potentially travel to your lungs and cause a life-threatening pulmonary embolism. Don't worry if you forget and find yourself rubbing a sore area without thinking, but try as best you can to resist the urge.

Pneumonia

TIP 575

BEWARE OF THE BIRDCAGE!

Parakeets and lovebirds can transmit psittacosis—a rare form of pneumonia commonly known as parrot fever—to their unsuspecting human owners. Sick birds can spread the infectious microorganism in dust from the feathers, in droppings, or even by biting a finger. Psitta-cosis symptoms include fever, chills, headaches, muscle aches, loss of appetite, nausea, vomiting, and enlarge-ment of the spleen.

Pneumonia

TIP 576

HOLD THE MUSTARD

Try a traditional mustard poultice to loosen the phlegm associat-ed with pneumonia. Mix dry mustard with enough warm water to make a thick paste. Spread the paste on thin cotton or cheese-cloth, fold, and place on your chest for several minutes. Don't overdo it: Mustard causes blistering if left on bare skin too long.

TIP *577*

THE PSA TEST

Doctors now can administer a blood test, called the PSA (prostate-specific antigen) test, to help detect prostate cancer. It is easy to give, relatively cheap, and has improved detection of early prostate cancer dramatically. Coupled with rectal exams and the newly developed KAI-1 genetic test, the PSA test enables doctors to detect and treat threatening prostate cancers at a very early stage. The American Cancer Society recommends that all men over 50 years of age have an annual PSA test; for information about a local screening site, call 1-800-ACS-2345.

TIP *578*

LIGHT THERAPY

Like other serious or chronic skin disorders, psoriasis may respond to light therapy, or phototherapy. Patients receive timed exposure to ultraviolet radiation, in some cases after taking an oral medication called psoralen. The treatment is repeated several times a week for up to eight sessions per month. Although many doctors and patients report positive results, the treatment can have serious short- and long-term side effects; the drug psoralen is not recommended for pregnant women, because of the potential risk to the developing fetus. While light therapy may not be right for every psoriasis sufferer, it may be worth discussing with your doctor.

TIP 579

THE CHICKWEED FACTOR

To relieve the itching of scabies, add a cup of oatmeal or cornstarch or a pinch of chickweed *(Stellaria media)* to your bath; soak in hot water and scrub with soap. Avoid overscrubbing, which can lead to a skin condition called eczematous scabies.

Shingles

TIP 580

SOOTHING SHINGLES

To cut down on the itching of shingles, ask your pharmacist to mix 78 percent calamine lotion with 20 percent rubbing alcohol, 1 percent phenol, and 1 percent menthol. You can apply this mixture continuously until your blisters scab over. Or try the Bach flower Rescue Remedy, applying the cream four times a day to relieve pain and inflammation.

Thyroid Problems

TIP 581

TAKE A STAND

For many people, the Shoulder Stand position, practiced at least once daily for 20 minutes, can help improve overall thyroid function.

Shoulder Stand

Lie on your back, hands at your sides. Lift both legs until they are at a right angle to your back. Supporting your hips with hands, inhale and extend your back and legs vertically. Slowly lower legs to release.

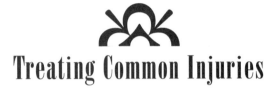

Treating Common Injuries

FIRST-AID

TECHNIQUES AND

AT-HOME REMEDIES

FOR BLISTERS, BRUISES,

BURNS, CUTS,

SPLINTERS, SPRAINS,

AND MANY OTHER

EVERYDAY BOO-BOOS

Treating Common Injuries

TIP *582*

BLACK AND BLUE AND ORANGES

If you bruise at the slightest pressure, it could indicate a vitamin C deficiency. Eat more oranges, broccoli, and sweet potatoes; the vitamin can also be taken in capsule form, but don't take high doses for prolonged periods.

TIP *583*

A PINEAPPLE A DAY MAKES THE BRUISE GO AWAY

Eating large amounts of pineapple or papaya can help wipe out a bruise. In addition to vitamin C, pineapples contain an enzyme, bromelain, that's believed to alter the chemistry of the blood, allowing it to be more easily reabsorbed by the body. Bromelain is also good for sore muscles and joints.

TIP *584*

THE COMFORT OF COMFREY

The herb comfrey *(Symphytum officinale)* can help clear up a bruise. Soak comfrey leaves in hot water, spread them on a cloth, and press the poultice to the bruise. Do not use if the skin is broken.

COMFREY

TIP *585*

IN THE BLINK OF AN EYE

Do not attempt to remove an object that is embedded in the eye. For a speck that is floating freely, pull the upper eyelid down over the lower one: This will create tears, which may wash out the object. If this does not work, but the object is visible on the surface of the eye or inside the lids, flush it out with water or lift it off with a damp cloth—not tissue or a cotton ball.

TIP *586*

FOR A BLEEDING NOSE

If your nose starts bleeding after a minor blow, lean your head forward, gently pinch both nostrils shut with your thumb and index finger, and hold for 10 minutes, breathing through your mouth. If this does not slow the bleeding, or if you feel blood going down your throat, see a doctor.

TIP *587*

OBJECT IN THE EAR

If something is stuck in your ear, tilt the ear down and try to shake it out. If this does not work, but the object is visible in the ear, a helper can try to remove it with tweezers. (Do not attempt this with a hard object, like a bead, or with an insect.) If the object refuses to budge, or if blood or fluids are draining from the ear, go to a hospital.

TIP*588*

A BUG IN YOUR EAR

If an insect crawls into your ear—and doesn't immediately crawl out—do not try to pull it out. Instead, put a dropperful of alcohol, oil, or vinegar into your ear canal to kill the invader, then flush it out with water.

TIP*589*

TRY A LITTLE TENDERNESS

For insect stings and bites of all sorts, apply ice to hold down swelling, then a paste of baking soda and water, salt and water, or —best of all—meat tenderizer.

TIP*590*

ITCH BUSTERS

An antihistamine can help with the itching and swelling of insect bites or stings. Aspirin or acetaminophen can relieve the pain. Or try homeopathic relief: for swelling, *Apis;* for itching, *Cantharis.*

TIP*591*

WHEN FIDO TURNS FIERCE

If your pet cat or dog takes a nip at you, you can treat the bite as you would any superficial cut. But if the wound is deep, or if it has been inflicted by a stray or wild animal that might be rabid, see your doctor.

TIP 592

FOR SLOPPY EATERS

If you've bitten your tongue, or burned it on too-hot food, hold
an ice cube in your mouth. In the following days, rinse frequently
with salt water or hydrogen peroxide, and avoid spicy foods.

TIP 593

BALM FOR BLISTERS

Blisters caused by new shoes or other friction against the skin can
be soothed with calendula *(Calendula officinalis)* ointment, vitamin E ointment or aloe cream. After the
blister breaks, cleanse the area with a mild antiseptic
such as hydrogen peroxide or calendula, and keep
it bandaged until the skin heals.

ALOE

TIP 594

LET IT BLEED

With minor cuts, it's a good idea to let the wound bleed a little,
since that will help remove debris and dirt from the tissue. If
bleeding persists for more than a few minutes, however, place a
clean cloth against the wound and press down on it, until the
blood flow is reduced.

TIP 595

A BLOOD-CHILLING
EXPERIENCE

If blood continues to trickle from a wound after pressure has
been applied, an ice pack—held against the skin for no more than
15 minutes—can cut off the flow by constricting blood vessels.

TIP 596

THE UNKINDEST CUTS

Some cuts need to be seen promptly by a doctor. Don't attempt
to treat a wound yourself if:

- The blood is spurting.
- You can see deep into the flesh.
- The cut is on the face, and you want to avoid a scar.
- The injury affects a joint.

TIP 597

CLEANING UP

When bleeding is under control, wash the wound thoroughly for
at least a minute with soap and water; then apply calendula *(Calendula officinalis)* ointment, hydrogen peroxide, or an antibacterial solution.

TIP 598

ANTIBIOTIC PROS & CONS

You can use over-the-counter antibiotic ointment for a laceration
or abrasion; loosely bandage the affected area after application.
But do not use ointment on deep puncture wounds; it can increase the likelihood of infection.

TIP *599*

ALL-PURPOSE HERB

To help heal burns, cuts and scrapes, blisters, sunburn, and frostbite, apply calendula *(Calendula officinalis)* ointment to
the injured skin. Herbalists consider this plant to be
one of the most effective treatments for minor wounds,
since it promotes healing, kills invasive bacteria, and by
numbing nerve endings provides pain relief.

CALENDULA

TIP *600*

A SWEET SOLUTION

Applied to a minor cut, honey can help prevent infection and
promote healing. Spread on a thin layer and cover with a loose
bandage; repeat daily.

TIP *601*

THE INS AND OUTS
OF VITAMIN E

The contents of a vitamin E capsule can be applied to the skin to
help with the healing of minor wounds; the vitamin is also good
for promoting healing if taken orally.

TIP *602*

BANDAID ASSISTANCE

To avoid pulling off a wound-protecting scab when you remove
a bandage, cut out the gauze center and lift it off, then gently remove the adhesive strips.

TIP *603*

MASSAGE AWAY SCAR TISSUE

To lessen potential scarring after a wound has healed, massage the skin with moisturizer.

TIP *604*

FOR A PAPER CUT

For relief from a paper cut, some people recommend applying a drop of a superstrength bonding glue. But you could end up gluing fingers together. Better to stick with something like calendula *(Calendula officinalis)* ointment, for healing and pain relief.

CALENDULA

TIP *605*

OF BURNING IMPORTANCE

The redness and tenderness of a first-degree burn—if it is not too widespread—can be treated at home. But get immediate medical help if:

- The burn was caused by electrical or chemical exposure.
- It is extremely painful.
- The skin looks white, or charred and black.
- An infection develops.

TIP *606*

COOL RELIEF

For a minor burn, hold the affected area under cool running water, then apply a cool—but not icy—compress.

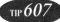

MILK, NOT BUTTER

Butter on a burn will hold in heat and encourage infection. Instead, try a milk compress, which can be particularly soothing.

IT ISN'T JUST
FOR HEMORRHOIDS

Preparation H—the hemorrhoid treatment—can help speed up healing of minor burns. Put a small amount on the affected area each day.

DON'T MESS WITH BLISTERS

Don't pop the blisters that erupt on burned skin; you'll end up with an infection worse than the original injury.

SUN SOAK

See a doctor if a sunburn is accompanied by fever, nausea, or extensive blistering. For minor burns, soak in a cool bath laced with several tablespoonfuls of baking soda, cornstarch, or cider vinegar, take aspirin, and drink plenty of fluids.

TIP *611*

FROST WARNING

Soak frost-bitten skin in a tub of warm water (101-104°F) for
about 45 minutes, or until feeling returns; then cover the area
with a cloth. Do not massage the skin. And whatever you do,
do not rub the area with snow.

TIP *612*

POISON CONTROL

If you think someone has injested poison, call your local poison
control center. (You should keep the number posted by your
phone.) Tell the center what chemical, household item, or plant
you suspect, and follow the instructions you are given. Do not
rely on the information on a label.

TIP *613*

A FAST RECOVERY
FROM POISONING

To rid your body of toxins after an episode of poisoning, drink
plenty of liquids, in particular fresh fruit and vegetable juices.
Solid food is probably best avoided for a day or two.
Also, try taking 15 drops of red clover *(Trifolium
pratense)* tincture twice a day.

RED CLOVER

TIP *614*

BEATING WHIPLASH

If a jolt leaves you with a sore neck, lie on your back on a firm
bed without a pillow. If the pain of whiplash persists for more
than a day, call your doctor.

TIP *615*

A PRESCRIPTION OF RICE

For the first two or three days after spraining or straining a limb, RICE—rest, ice, compression, and elevation—is the standard treatment. An ice pack—alternating 10 minutes on, 10 minutes off for a few hours each day for the first couple of days—will reduce inflammation. Elastic bandages will compress the area and alleviate swelling. And keeping the injured area elevated will promote drainage of fluid.

TIP *616*

KEEP AWAY FROM HEAT

Heating pads can be used to stimulate circulation and ease soreness after an injury. But don't use heat on swollen tissues; it will increase inflammation.

TIP *617*

BONE UP ON VINEGAR

To help a fracture mend, increase your intake of minerals, such as calcium, magnesium, boron and, in particular, silica. Apple cider vinegar is an abundant source of silica: Take 1 tsp in a cup of warm water or juice three times a day. Another good source of silica is horsetail *(Equisetum arvense);* consult an herbalist for dosage.

HORSETAIL

TIP *618*

THE LOW-DOWN ON
LOWER-BACK PAIN

Two or three days of bed rest are recommended for strained lower-back muscles. Put a pillow beneath your knees to take pressure off your back.

TIP *619*

SPRAIN RELIEF

For the two or three weeks it takes a typical sprain or strain to heal, aspirin or ibuprofen can help reduce inflammation and pain.

TIP *620*

THE MANY USES OF ARNICA

Homeopaths prescribe *Arnica* for the pain and swelling of sprains and strains. It can be taken orally or applied as a salve. It is also recommended for fractures; if taken immediately, it can help prevent shock.

TIP *621*

SPICE UP YOUR
MEDICINE CABINET

Capsaicin, the active ingredient in chili peppers, can help numb the pain of injured joints or muscles. Ointments and oils containing capsaicin are available at drugstores and herbal stores. But this is strong medicine, and it is best used under a doctor's supervision.

TIP *622*

TURNING AROUND
TENNIS ELBOW

A mild case of tennis elbow might benefit from what's called the counterstrain technique. Get someone to rotate your arm in the direction opposite from the one that causes you pain; hold that position for 90 seconds. Repeat several times a day.

TIP *623*

SOAK OUT A SPLINTER

Before you try to extract a splinter, soak the area where it is embedded for 15 minutes in hot water. Sometimes this will make the splinter come out on its own.

TIP *624*

PROBING INVESTIGATIONS

If you do have to dig out a splinter, first numb the area with an ice cube, then douse it with hydrogen peroxide. Sterilize a pair of flat-ended tweezers with alcohol, and probe carefully. After the splinter has been removed, wash the skin thoroughly and apply an antiseptic ointment such as calendula *(Calendula officinalis)*.

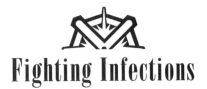

Fighting Infections

Natural Remedies

AND THE BEST

CONVENTIONAL

TREATMENTS

TO HELP YOU

BEAT BACK INFECTIONS

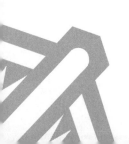

Fighting Infections

TIP 625

WASH YOUR HANDS!

It's not just the smart thing socially: Keeping your hands clean can help keep you healthy. Killing germs on skin requires more than a quick rinse, though; you need to really scrub with soap. And you need to do it many times a day, particularly if you're around people with colds.

TIP 626

THE COLD WAR

If begun at the moment you suspect that a cold is imminent, alternative treatments can often reduce the intensity and duration of the illness.

- Place peppermint *(Mentha piperita)* or eucalyptus *(Eucalyptus globulus)* leaves or oil in a bowl, add boiling water, drape a towel over your head and breathe the vapors. If the vapor temperature is 110°, it can kill cold-causing germs on contact.
- Take echinacea *(Echinacea* spp.), available in capsules; the herb stimulates the immune system, enhancing resistance to infection.
- Garlic *(Allium sativum)* also boosts immune response. If you feel that you can handle hearty foods, you can simply add fresh garlic to soups, stews, and pasta sauces. Otherwise, take three garlic capsules three times a day.
- For a sore throat, suck on zinc lozenges or gargle with a calendula *(Calendula officinalis)* tincture.
- Megadoses of vitamin C cannot prevent colds, but they may help lessen the severity of symptoms.

TIP *627*

COLD SYMPTOMS: BE SPECIFIC

Conventional medicine offers many cold treatments. Some are best avoided. Multi-ingredient "cold and flu" preparations are likely to contain inadequate doses of the medications you need to effectively treat your symptoms, while drugging you for symptoms you do not have. So it's better to pick medicines that target your specific problems, rather than taking the shotgun approach.

- Decongestants—pill or spray—can ease congestion, though they should be used only for a few days.
- Coughing, since it helps to expel mucus and germs, should probably not be suppressed, but if your cough interferes with sleep, try an over-the-counter cough medicine containing dextromethorphan.
- Some researchers believe that taking aspirin to lower the fever that accompanies a cold is counterproductive: Your body may be using heat to kill the virus. Aspirin—and acetaminophen—may also worsen congestion. Instead, use ibuprofen for aches and pains. But if the fever is more than 102.6°, you do need aspirin or acetaminophen. (Never give a child aspirin.)

TIP *628*

SLEEPING IT OFF

Since neither conventional nor alternative methods can cure a cold—only your immune system can do that—the most important thing is to let your system heal itself. Sleep is crucial. Follow your body's cues; if it wants 12 hours a night, that's what you should give it. Keep yourself well hydrated by drinking 6 to 10 glasses of water each day, and use a cool-air vaporizer at night to help keep your tissues from drying out.

TIP *629*

VIRAL AVOIDANCE

You can take steps to avoid catching colds. Regular, moderate
exercise seems to strengthen the immune system. Eat a balanced
diet, and supplement it to make up for any deficiencies. Cut
down on stimulants such as sugar, coffee, and other caffeinated
products. Don't smoke. Minimize contact with people with
colds. Wash your hands thoroughly and frequently. There's also
evidence that the heat of a sauna may prevent cold germs from
reproducing, so if possible, visit a sauna twice a week.

TIP *630*

VOICING CONCERN

A cold virus can cause an inflammation of the larynx, causing you
to become hoarse or lose your voice. (Overuse of the vocal cords
can have the same effect.) If you have laryngitis, try not to talk
at all, drink plenty of liquids, and apply warm compresses to your throat. Herbal remedies include gargling
with teas made from ginger *(Zingiber officinale)*, red
sage *(Salvia officinalis* var. *rubia)*, mayberry *(Myrica* spp.)
or white oak *(Quercus alba)*. If your voice does not return
in a week, see your doctor; you might have a bacterial
complication that requires antibiotics.

SAGE

TIP *631*

FIGHTING THE FLU

If you come down with the flu, aromatherapists recommend
adding 2 drops of tea tree *(Melaleuca* spp.) oil to a hot bath to
help your immune system fight the viral infection and ease your
symptoms. Tea tree oil can be irritating to the skin, however, so
don't use more than 2 drops in a full bath.

TIP 632

SINUSITIS IS A PAIN

Sinusitis is an infection of the cavities that flank the eyes and nose. Symptoms include difficulty breathing, postnasal drip, and a feeling of pressure behind the eyes. To rid yourself of sinusitis, you need to restore proper drainage. Try applying warm compresses, inhaling the steam from clove or ginger tea, doing acupressure, or using a homeopathic nasal spray, which can clear congestion without side effects. If sinuses do not open up in a week, see a doctor, who will prescribe antibiotics, decongestants, or inhaled steroids.

Large Intestine 20
Using your index or middle fingers, press hard on the outer edge of the nostrils at the base of the nose.

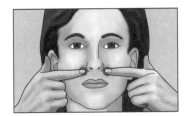

TIP 633

VANQUISHING STREP

Since the flu usually begins with a day or two of feeling not quite right, the sudden development of an excruciatingly sore throat and a high fever—particularly when there is no congestion—may signal the bacterial infection known as strep throat. Since strep can lead to more serious illnesses, you should quickly go to a doctor, who will be able to cure the infection with antibiotics. Make sure to finish your prescription; prematurely discontinuing treatment can make the disease come back in a more virulent form. Take acidophilus capsules, 1 capsule twice a day, to replace important intestinal flora killed by the antibiotics, and take 1,000 mg of vitamin C, twice a day, to help support your immune system.

TIP *634*

EASING BRONCHITIS

Just when a cold or flu seems to be on the wane, it starts: a hacking cough, a profusion of phlegm, tightness in the chest. You've got bronchitis, an inflammation of the lungs usually caused by a viral infection. Mild cases generally don't require professional medical treatment; the problem should clear up with a week of rest and steam therapy. You can also try an infusion of coltsfoot (*Tussilago farfara*), which may relax bronchial-tube spasms. If you're not better in a week, if the cough interferes with sleep, or if your mucus increases in thickness and volume, see a doctor; you may have pneumonia, a potentially fatal infection.

TIP *635*

GETTING THINGS OUT OF YOUR CHEST

Try to clear the lungs of phlegm and other fluids, which is essential for recovery from infections like bronchitis and pneumonia:

- Massage the upper back with a lotion that contains a few drops of eucalyptus (*Eucalyptus globulus*) oil.
- Try an herbal expectorant: Combine 2 oz licorice (*Glycyrrhiza glabra*), 1 oz wild black cherry (*Prunus serotina*), 1 oz coltsfoot (*Tussilago farfara*), ⅛ oz lobelia (*Lobelia inflata*), and 1 oz horehound (*Marrubium vulgare*). Simmer 1 tbsp in a cup of water for five minutes; let steep for 10 minutes, strain and drink every two hours.
- Use a mustard poultice: Mix dry mustard with enough warm water to make a thick paste, spread on a cloth, and place on your chest for a few minutes.
- Inhale steam that contains pine (*Pinus sylvestris*), lavender (*Lavandula officinalis*), or ginger (*Zingiber officinale*).
- Try the homeopathic remedy *Spongia* or *Hepar sulphuris;* consult a homeopathic practitioner.

TIP *636*

HARD TO STOMACH

Sometimes known as the stomach flu, gastroenteritis is a general term for a number of intestinal upsets, from viral or bacterial infections to food poisoning. Unless the cramps, nausea, and vomiting last more than a couple of days or are accompanied by high fever, you can treat gastroenteritis at home. Rest, drink plenty of liquids, and when your appetite is back eat bland foods like rice and bananas. Yogurt, since it helps restore healthy intestinal bacteria, is particularly helpful. Or try a tea made with meadowsweet *(Filipendula ulmaria)* or ginger *(Zingiber officinale)* to ease nausea.

Tea: *Pour 1 cup boiling water on 2 tsp dried meadowsweet, steep for 15 minutes; drink three times daily.*

TIP *637*

BYPASS DIVERTICULITIS

A pain on the left side of the abdomen could be a sign of diverticulitis, an infection of the pouches that can form along the walls of the intestine. A potentially serious condition, it can lead to internal bleeding if left untreated. If caught early, before abcesses develop and other organs are involved, diverticulitis may require only bed rest, a liquid diet, stool softeners, antibiotics, and antispasmodics; a complementary treatment for a mild case involves massaging the lower abdomen with circular clockwise strokes, then drinking a cup of chamomile *(Matricaria recutita)* tea. To help prevent diverticulitis, eat a high-fiber diet and avoid refined foods.

CHAMOMILE

TIP 638

THE ACID TEST FOR ULCERS

Contrary to what doctors believed for decades, it seems that a bad diet or stress is not the primary cause of the perforations of the stomach lining known as ulcers; instead, the majority of cases may be caused by infection with the *Helicobacter pylori* bacterium (though heavy alcohol use, smoking, too much aspirin, and stress can be contributing factors). If you experience burning upper abdominal pain that is relieved by antacids, you should be evaluated by a doctor. If the cause is bacterial, you will be given antibiotics, as well as medications that can help minimize stomach-acid secretion. As for what you can do on your own, since stress can cause acid overload, you can try stress-management techniques such as meditation, deep breathing, guided imagery, and yoga.

TIP 639

DIGESTING INFORMATION
ABOUT THE PANCREAS

Though it is most often the result of excessive alcohol consumption, pancreatitis—inflammation of the gland that produces insulin and digestive enzymes—can be the result of an infection. Pancreatitis is a serious condition, so consult a doctor immediately if you experience sudden, intense pains in the middle of your abdomen, or abdominal tenderness along with fever and a rapid pulse. Once the acute problem has been solved, you can use alternative methods to prevent further attacks. A combination of glycerates of fringe-tree bark *(Chionanthus virginicus)*, balmony *(Chelone glabra)*, and milk thistle *(Silybum marianum)* may help promote fat digestion; take 1 tsp of the mixture three times daily. Chromium supplements, MILK THISTLE   300 mcg daily, can stabilize blood sugar levels.

TIP *640*

ELIMINATING
KIDNEY INFECTIONS

Kidney infections, which are caused by *E. coli* bacteria, usually begin as bladder infections, although they can also be triggered by the use of catheters. They are a serious problem, requiring immediate medical attention. See your doctor if you experience painful urination or notice blood in your urine. Treatment is fairly simple: Resting, taking antibiotics, and drinking 6 to 10 glasses of fluid daily will usually bring the infection under control within 48 hours. Until you are cured, avoid irritating foods such as alcohol, coffee, caffeinated colas and teas, salt, chocolate, vinegar, citrus fruits, and spicy dishes.

TIP *641*

STARVING A CHRONIC
YEAST CONDITION

Some doctors—though by no means all—believe that patients exhibiting a variety of vague, difficult-to-diagnose complaints may be suffering from chronic yeast infection. The treatment for this condition is primarily dietary: People are advised to stay away from dairy foods, red meat, pork, beans, bread and other yeast products, foods containing vinegar, sugar, alcohol, and sweets. In addition, systemic antifungal drugs are sometimes prescribed. Pau d'arco *(Tabebuia impetiginosa)* tea may have the same systemic effect. Tea made from barberry *(Berberis vulgaris)* may also help.

TIP 642

OUTGROWING YEAST INFECTIONS

A fungal organism that thrives in the mouth, gastrointestinal tract, and genitalia, *Candida albicans* is usually held in check by helpful bacteria. But when an illness, stress, or antibiotic therapy throws off the fungus-bacteria balance, the result is one of a number of yeast infections: moniliasis (in the vagina), balanitis (in the penis), thrush (in the mouth or esophagus), athlete's foot (between the toes). Moniliasis and athlete's foot can generally be treated with over-the-counter remedies or tea tree oil (*Melaleuca* spp.); thrush, which is marked by painless white patches in the mouth and throat, requires prescription antifungal medication. An herbal alternative is to gargle with calendula (*Calendula officinalis*) tincture or drink 3 cups of pau d'arco (*Tabebuia impetiginosa*) tea every day.

TEA TREE

TIP 643

FACING UP TO IMPETIGO

A skin problem that can be caused by staph or by the strep bacterium is impetigo, patches of blisters, usually on the face, that become red and oozy, then harden into a yellow crust. Mild cases of impetigo may clear up after a couple of days of washing with an antibacterial soap or a goldenseal (*Hydrastis canadensis*) paste. If the sores persist, see your doctor, who will prescribe an antibiotic ointment. (Do not use over-the-counter antibiotic creams; they are too weak and may spread the infection.) Since impetigo is highly contagious, someone with the infection should have his own bar of soap and his own towels, which should be washed separately.

Paste: *Mix 1 tbsp goldenseal with enough water or egg white to make a paste; apply it to your sores, which should clear in two to three days.*

TIP *644*

SHAVING FACE

A generally harmless bacterium, *Staphylococcus aureus* can cause a multitude of disorders if it enters the body through a break in the skin. One common problem is folliculitis, a superficial infection of the hair follicles that primarily affects men who shave. Men who are prone to outbreaks of the small, white-headed pustules should wash their faces with an antibacterial soap before shaving, use a razor that's been soaked in rubbing alcohol, and apply an antibacterial skin cream when they're finished.

TIP *645*

THE BOILING POINT

When staph penetrates deep into a hair follicle, the result is the large, pus-filled inflammation known as a boil. Do not squeeze or attempt to lance a boil; instead, wash the area with antibacterial soap, use compresses of warm water laced with Epsom salts, and apply antibiotic ointment. Or you can try various herbal remedies, such as topical tea tree oil (*Melaleuca* spp.), a poutice of slippery elm *(Ulmus fulva)*, or a wash of goldenseal *(Hydrastis canadensis)* mixed with calendula *(Calendula officinalis)* tincture or distilled witch hazel. After the boil breaks and drains—this usually takes about two weeks—cover it with a bandage.

GOLDENSEAL

TIP *646*

THE RED LINE ON BOILS

Some boils require more than home care. See a doctor if a boil is extremely painful; if it is located on the face or spine; or if it does not clear up in a reasonable period of time. Most important of all, get immediate help for a boil that has red lines radiating from it or is accompanied by a fever; this could indicate that blood poisoning has set in.

TIP *647*

SHINGLES:
AN ELDERLY INFECTION

Anyone who has ever had chickenpox continues to harbor the virus in the nerve cells of the spine. It may lie dormant your whole life. But particularly among the elderly, an illness or physical or emotional trauma can reactivate it and cause an eruption of painful blisters known as shingles. There is no cure, but antiviral drugs can limit the spread of the rash, and corticosteroids can reduce inflammation. Some home remedies can also help ease the discomfort. Crush two aspirin, mix them with 2 tbsp rubbing alcohol, and apply the paste to lesions three times a day to desensitize nerve endings. Ask your pharmacist to mix 78 percent calamine lotion with 1 percent phenol, 1 percent menthol, and 20 percent rubbing alcohol and apply the mixture to ease itching. A commercially prepared gel made from a licorice extract may interfere with virus growth. Ice—10 minutes on, 5 minutes off—can be soothing.

TIP *648*

OUT ON A LIMB

An infection of a wound is one of the causes of phlebitis, a condition in which a vein in the leg becomes red and tender. Cases of superficial phlebitis can be treated by wearing elastic support stockings, resting with the leg elevated 6 to 12 inches above the level of the heart, applying hot compresses, and taking aspirin. (Resist the temptation to massage the aching area, since this could dislodge a blood clot.) If symptoms do not dissipate within 10 days, or if the entire limb is swollen and painful, see a doctor. You may have deep phlebitis, which will require treatment with antibiotics and antiocoagulants.

TIP *649*

ICING DOWN A COLD SORE

Cold sores, also known as fever blisters, are caused by the highly contagious herpes virus. As soon as you feel the tingling that precedes the development of a cold sore, apply a water-based zinc ointment. Once the sore has sprouted, you can soothe the discomfort with ice, over-the-counter medicines that contain the numbing agent phenol, or a doctor-prescribed anesthetic gel. To help heal a cold sore, apply witch hazel; extracts of nettle *(Urtica dioica)*, goldenseal *(Hydrastis canadensis)*, or myrrh *(Commiphora molmol)*; or tea tree *(Melaleuca* spp.) or vitamin E oil. If you touch your sore, don't touch any other part of your body until you've washed your hands thoroughly; you could end up with herpes of the eyes or genitals. And no kissing until the sore is gone.

NETTLE

TIP *650*

FEELING DOWN IN THE MOUTH?

Canker sores are annoying infections of the inside of the mouth, usually lasting about a week, that afflict half of Americans in any year. The cause is not known, but many researchers suspect that dietary deficiencies, food allergies, and stress play a role. If you're prone to developing the sores, avoid coffee, spices, and acidic foods; brush your teeth with baking soda; and take supplements of vitamin C, B complex, folic acid, iron, and zinc. To treat a canker sore, rinse your mouth four times a day with a combination of 2 oz hydrogen peroxide, 2 oz water, and 1 tsp each of salt and baking soda, or use a drugstore ointment that contains glycerin and peroxide.

TIP 651

ALL GUMMED UP

Periodontal disease is an infection of the gums that afflicts almost all Americans over the age of 60. The earliest stage of the infection is gingivitis, in which pockets filled with bacteria form at the gum line, causing painless inflammation, swelling, and redness. If the pockets deepen, the result is periodontitis, an inflammation of the ligaments that hold teeth in their sockets; periodontitis can cause tooth loss. The best treatment for gum disease is prevention—regular

MYRRH visits to the dentist along with thorough daily brushing and flossing. Mouthwashes can also help; try a mixture of bayberry (*Myrica* spp.) and prickly ash *(Zanthoxylum americanum)*, or sage *(Salvia officinalis)* and chamomile *(Matricaria recutita)*. Massaging your gums with goldenseal *(Hydrastis canadensis)* or myrrh *(Commiphora molmol)* is also beneficial.

TIP 652

LYME DISEASE

Caused by a bacterium that is spread by deer ticks, Lyme disease can be difficult to diagnose, since many of its symptoms resemble those of the flu. The one definitive sign of infection is an expanding bull's-eye rash, although this does not always occur. See your doctor promptly if you develop the rash; if you suddenly develop knee pain or swelling unrelated to an injury; or if flulike symptoms develop after a camping trip, particularly if you were bitten by a tick. To protect yourself from the disease-carrying tick, wear long sleeves and long pants tucked into socks, and put insect repellent around your ankles. Once you're indoors, check yourself for ticks, and remove any you find with tweezers.

TIP *653*

SPOTTING ROCKY
MOUNTAIN SPOTTED FEVER

Like Lyme disease, Rocky Mountain Spotted Fever is a potentially serious, difficult-to-diagnose illness spread by ticks. In RMSF,
the rash consists of very small pinkish spots that show up first on
the wrists or ankles, then spread to the torso. Accompanying the
rash—which generally begins three to 10 days after the tick bite—
are flulike symptoms. As is the case with Lyme disease, early antibiotic treatment is essential; the longer you delay seeing the
doctor, the greater the chance of permanent damage or death.

TIP *654*

LOCKING OUT TETANUS

One of the most dangerous microbial poisons is a spore found in
soil, house dust, and animal or human excrement. If this spore
enters the body through a wound, the result can be tetanus, a
condition in which the muscles lock up, making it impossible to
breathe. If you are wounded by an object that has been in contact
with soil—even if the wound barely bleeds—cleanse the cut thoroughly, and see a doctor within 24 hours. The doctor will cut
away any damaged tissue and give you a tetanus shot if you have
not had one recently. (You should get a booster every 10 years.)

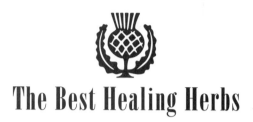

The Best Healing Herbs

An ALPHABETICAL

GUIDE TO

THE MOST

EFFECTIVE HERBAL

REMEDIES—FROM

ALFALFA TO YARROW

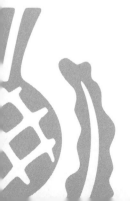

The Best Healing Herbs

Alfalfa

TIP 655

AN INTERIOR CLEANSER

Effective as a body cleanser, alfalfa *(Medicago sativa)* treats bladder inflammation, bloating, indigestion, constipation, and even bad breath. Add sprouts to salads and sandwiches, or drink 3 cups a day of alfalfa tea.

Tea: Steep 1 to 2 tsp of dried leaves per cup of water for five to 10 minutes.

Aloe

TIP 656

NOT JUST FOR BURNS

Add 1 or 2 cups of aloe gel to a warm bath to relieve the pain and itch of sunburn or skin lesions, or apply the gel directly to minor burns, sunburned skin, chickenpox lesions, poison ivy rashes, and other irritations. The juice of the *Aloe barbadensis* plant contains several ingredients that have been shown to reduce inflammation.

Black Cohosh

TIP 657

ESPECIALLY FOR WOMEN

Relieve menopausal and menstrual discomforts, including premenstrual stress, with the root and rhizome of black cohosh *(Cimicifuga racemosa)*, which acts like estrogen in the body. The herb is available over-the-counter as a tincture or syrup, in capsules, and as a fluid extract. Because it can cause serious side effects, black cohosh should be taken only under medical supervision.

Boneset

TIP 658

THE NATURAL WAY
TO BRING DOWN A FEVER

Drink an infusion of boneset *(Eupatorium perfoliatum)* to cool
fevers that accompany colds and flu. Drink it as hot as you
can, no more than a cup every half hour, up to 4 cups in
six hours; don't take more than 6 cups in a 24-hour period. You'll want to mix it with an herbal tea or add plenty
of lemon and honey to mask the bitter taste.

> **Infusion:** *Pour 1 cup of boiling water onto 2 to 3 tsp of the
> dried herb and let it steep for 15 minutes.*

Burdock

TIP 659

GOOD INSIDE AND OUT

Treat genital and urinary tract irritations with a decoction of burdock *(Arctium lappa)* root, available in sliced form
over the counter. The tea also speeds healing of skin
wounds and ulcers; soak a clean cloth in the solution
and place it on the affected area.

> **Tea:** *Boil 1 tsp of the root in 3 cups of water for 30 minutes,
> and drink up to 3 cups a day.*

Calendula

TIP 660

SAVIOR OF THE SKIN

A natural antiseptic and anti-inflammatory agent, calendula
(Calendula officinalis) is one of the best herbs for treating wounds, skin abrasions, and infections. Rub calendula ointment on cuts, chickenpox or measles lesions,
any eruptive skin disease, diaper rash, athlete's foot,
and burns. Use the tincture for sore throats and colds.

Cayenne

TIP 661

PEP UP WITH PEPPER

Available in powder form, cayenne *(Capsicum annuum* var. *annuum)* is an effective energy booster, thanks to the natural stimulant capsaicin.

Infusion: Pour a cup of boiling water over ½ to 1 tsp powder and steep for 10 minutes. Mix 1 tbsp of the infusion with hot water and drink as needed.

Chamomile

TIP 662

SWEET DREAMS

At bedtime, a cup of tea brewed with the flowers of German chamomile *(Matricaria recutita)* can calm the central nervous system and speed you to slumber. The same brew also soothes indigestion, stomach cramps, gas, and ulcers. Drink 1 cup up to four times a day, but beware that too much can cause diarrhea.

Tea: Pour 8 oz boiling water over 2 tsp chamomile flowers and steep for 10 minutes.

Chaste Tree

TIP 663

A HORMONAL BALANCING ACT

The compounds found in berries of the chaste tree *(Vitex agnus-castus)* bring the female sex hormones, estrogen and progesterone, into balance and can be used to treat menstrual irregularities, premenstrual stress, and endometriosis, as well as to promote lactation in breastfeeding mothers and prevent early miscarriage that may result from hormonal imbalances.

Tea: Pour 1 cup boiling water onto 1 tsp ripe berries and let it stand for 10 to 15 minutes. Drink three times a day.

Coltsfoot

TIP 664

COUGH SUPPRESSANT AND EXPECTORANT

Soothe your cough with three hot cups per day of tea brewed with coltsfoot *(Tussilago farfara)*. **Warning:** Use coltsfoot only as prescribed by a practitioner, for short periods of time, and do not give it to children under the age of two, pregnant or nursing women, alcoholics, or anyone with liver disease.

> *Tea: Steep 1 to 3 tsp of dried flowers or leaves in a cup of boiling-hot water for 10 minutes.*

Comfrey

TIP 665

EXTERNAL USE ONLY

For sprains, strains, cuts, insect bites, bruises, and skin ulcers and inflammations, sprinkle a powder of dried comfrey *(Symphytum officinale)* on the area and cover with a clean cloth. Comfrey contains allantoin, which fosters the growth of new cells. Herbalists recommend against using comfrey internally or if you are pregnant.

Dandelion

TIP 666

THE GOOD WEED

Use dandelion *(Taraxacum officinale)* as a diuretic to relieve symptoms associated with high blood pressure, premenstrual syndrome, menstrual pain, and joint pain. The plant also provides a nutritional boost, with rich supplies of antioxidant vitamins A and C, as well as potassium—a mineral typically lost when using diuretics. Drink up to 4 cups of tea per day, or simply toss a few fresh leaves in your salad.

> *Tea: Steep 1 tbsp dried or 2 tbsp fresh leaves in 8 oz boiling-hot water for 10 minutes.*

Echinacea

TIP 667

GARDEN-VARIETY ANTIBIOTIC

A popular garden plant, echinacea (*Echinacea* spp.) fights many types of bacterial and viral infection by bolstering the immune system's white blood cells in their battle against foreign invaders. Take the herb, available over the counter in the form of tea, capsules, and tincture, for colds, flu, respiratory illnesses, mononucleosis, ear infections, blood poisoning, and bladder infections.

Eyebright

TIP 668

THE EYES HAVE IT

For itching, red, or tearing eyes due to allergies, colds, or conjunctivitis, apply a compress of the aptly named herb eyebright (*Euphrasia officinalis*) for 15 minutes, a few times a day. *Compress: Boil 1 to 2 tbsp dried eyebright in a pint of water for 10 minutes; after the water cools, strain out the herbs, dip a sterile cloth in the fluid and wring it out, then place it on your eyes.*

Feverfew

TIP 669

FOR MIGRAINE RELIEF

Take 85 mg of feverfew (*Chrysanthemum parthenium*) in capsule or pill form every day to stave off migraine headaches. The leaves contain parthenolide, a chemical that blocks the release of inflammatory substances in the blood that are believed to trigger migraine onset. You may need to take the herb for two or three months before you notice an effect.

Garlic

TIP 670

THE LOVE BULB

Allium sativum—everyday garlic—helps alleviate digestive and intestinal disorders, and may also be used to strengthen the cardiovascular system by lowering blood pressure and reducing cholesterol. It's available in tablet form, but if you love the flavor, keep a bulb in stock in your kitchen. Add a clove or two to vegetable and meat dishes and sauces, or press it into your salad dressing. Or drizzle a little olive oil over a whole garlic bulb, wrap it in foil, and roast it in the oven for an hour; the individual cloves, which lose their acrid pungency in the oven, are delicious when spread on slices of whole wheat bread.

Ginger

TIP 671

QUELLING THE QUEASIES

A cup of ginger tea, made with the dried root of *Zingiber officinale,* soothes motion sickness, morning sickness, and other digestive upsets by way of gingerols, which calm the abdomen and relieve excess gas. Inhale ginger steam to ease sinusitis or upper-respiratory congestion; gargle for sore throat relief.

> **Tea:** *Boil 1 oz dried root in 1 cup water for 15 to 20 minutes.*

TIP 672

HERBAL BRAIN FOOD

One of the most important benefits of *Ginkgo biloba* is its ability to improve blood flow throughout the body, including the brain. Use over-the-counter capsules or tincture to improve mental concentration, reduce emotional fatigue and depression, and treat vertigo and ringing in the ears. Ginkgo's ability to expand blood vessels also makes it an effective treatment for phlebitis and leg ulcers; for these serious conditions, use ginkgo under a medical professional's care.

TIP 673

A CUP OF PREVENTION

Bolster your immune system and increase your resistance to colds, flu, and exhaustion with a daily cup of tea made from the root of Siberian ginseng *(Eleutherococcus senticosus)*, a more subtle and less dangerous cousin of the Asian and American varieties. Or you can use over-the-counter tablets, capsules, prepared teas, and even cured rock candy.

Tea: *Boil 1 oz fresh root in 1 cup water for 15 to 20 minutes.*

Goldenseal

TIP 674

GOOD AS GOLD

Treat a sore throat or sinusitis with the roots and rhizomes of goldenseal *(Hydrastis canadensis)*, which dries up secretions, reduces inflammation, and fights infection in mucous membranes. Drink goldenseal tea three times a day; a compress dampened with the solution and applied to the skin can also help clear up eczema and other rashes. Another choice is to take 15 drops of glycerated tincture two or three times a day.

> **Tea:** *Pour a cupful of boiling water over 2 tsp of the herb, available in bulk over the counter, and let it steep for 15 minutes.*

Gotu Kola

TIP 675

FATIGUE FIGHTER

Gotu kola *(Centella asiatica)* is an excellent choice for chronic fatigue and for stimulating the adrenal glands. Take 15 drops of glycerated tincture in the morning and the afternoon for three or four weeks to recharge your system. You can also use gotu kola for some skin problems. Soak a cotton pad in diluted tincture, and place it over burns, cuts, patches of psoriasis, or any other skin inflammation or injury to soothe and promote healing. But start with a weak solution and increase the concentration as necessary; the herb itself may cause a secondary rash if used too much, too soon.

Hawthorn ● TIP *676*

FOR YOUR HEART—SOMETIMES

Herbalists use the flowers, fruit, and leaves of the hawthorn *(Crataegus laevigata* or *C. oxyacantha)* for remedies that serve as a mild heart tonic. Some practitioners think the plant may also have a calming effect and prescribe it for insomnia. But you should always use this herb under the supervision of a healthcare practitioner; hawthorn has dangerous side effects, including dramatic drops in blood pressure.

Hops ● TIP *677*

AN HERB WITH A PAST

An ingredient of beer for more than a thousand years, hops *(Humulus lupulus)* has an even longer history as a sedative. For general anxiety, drink up to 3 cups a day of brewed tea. You can also soothe an acid stomach and aid digestion by drinking it cold an hour before mealtimes or just after eating.

Tea: Brew 2 tsp dried herb per cup of boiling water; steep for 15 minutes.

Horsetail ● TIP *678*

RINSE AWAY BLADDER INFLAMMATION

A cold cup of horsetail *(Equisetum arvense)* tea four times a day can help clear up bladder infections and urethritis by increasing the production of urine, flushing infection out of the system. The herb is also good for strengthening nails, skin, and hair, and for helping to heal bone fractures.

Tea: Steep 2 tsp of dried horsetail in 8 oz of boiling-hot water for 15 minutes, or use 1 tbsp of the fresh herb. Both are available over the counter.

Kelp

TIP 679

HELP FROM KELP

Rich in iodide, kelp *(Fucus* spp.) is a natural treatment for goiter and low thyroid, which is can be caused by a deficiency of the element. Take capsules, or drink an infusion three times a day.

Infusion: *Place 2 to 3 tsp dried or powdered kelp in a cup of boiling water.*

Lavender

TIP 680

LAVENDER BLUES

The spicy, energizing aroma of lavender *(Lavandula officinalis* or *L. angustifolia)* can stimulate mental processes and help alleviate depression, especially when it is combined with rosemary. Add a few drops of the essential oil to a warm bath and relax into it.

Licorice

TIP 681

ON THE SPOT REMEDY

For herpes sores and other skin inflammations, try sprinkling a little licorice powder on the spot. The *Glycyrrhiza glabra* plant is often used as an external antibiotic to speed healing.

Lobelia

TIP 682

EASING MUSCLE STRAIN

If you've strained a muscle, apply a compress of *Lobelia inflata*, which acts as a relaxant to ease the discomfort. Avoid using lobelia internally unless you're being supervised by a health-care practitioner because of potentially dangerous side effects.
Compress: Steep ¼ to ½ tsp of dried herb in 1 cup boiling water for 10 to 15 minutes; soak a piece of cloth in the warm infusion, wring it out, and drape over the muscle.

Marsh Mallow

TIP 683

MELLOW THE BABY
WITH MALLOW

Dot a gel of marsh mallow *(Althaea officinalis)*, made by mixing a few drops of water with some finely chopped marsh mallow root, on the sore gums of teething babies and toddlers. The healing substance in the plant is mucilage, which is particularly soothing to inflamed mucous membranes such as tissues in the mouth; it is safe for babies in low doses.

Milk Thistle

TIP 684

LIVER LOVER

Silymarin, the active ingredient in the seeds of milk thistle *(Silybum marianum)*, is thought to prompt the growth of healthy new liver cells and to increase the liver's stock of important detoxifying agents. For liver problems, including cirrhosis and hepatitis, or just to keep the vital organ in top shape, eat a teaspoon of freshly ground seeds up to three times a day.

Mullein

TIP *685*

AN HERBAL EXPECTORANT

Boil fresh leaves of mullein *(Verbascum thapsus)* and inhale
the steam to treat coughs and congestion. Use caution, though: Pregnant or nursing women and people
with a history of cancer should not take mullein, and no
one should ingest the seeds, which are toxic.

Myrrh

TIP *686*

DOWN IN THE MOUTH

Gargling or rinsing with a mouthwash containing myrrh *(Commiphora molmol)* can help heal gum disease, sore throats,
and other mouth infections. Myrrh fights infection by
stimulating the production of white blood cells and
by direct antibacterial action.

> ***Mouthwash:*** *Steep 1 tsp of the powdered herb and 1 tsp
> boric acid in a pint of boiling water, let it stand 30 min-
> utes, strain, and use when it has cooled.*

Nettle

TIP *687*

NETTLED BY ARTHRITIS?

Ease the symptoms of arthritis with capsules or a prepared tincture of nettle *(Urtica dioica),* which functions as a
diuretic and flushes toxins out of the body. If you
take nettle regularly, be sure to eat plenty of foods
high in potassium, such as bananas and fresh vegetables, because the herb's diuretic action will deplete
you of this essential nutrient.

Parsley

TIP *688*

NOT JUST ANOTHER
PRETTY GARNISH

There's more than one good reason to eat that sprig of parsley *(Petroselinum crispum)* on your dinner plate: Its ability to ease muscle spasms and cramps helps calm indigestion; it can help treat bladder infections; it provides a generous dose of vitamins C and A; and it's a natural breath freshener. Eat up!

Passionflower

TIP *689*

CALMING PASSION

Pleasant-tasting passionflower *(Passiflora incarnata)*, thought to have a sedating effect on the central nervous system, may help on that occasional sleepless night. Take a dropperful of tincture in warm water at bedtime. Passionflower does have serious side effects if used improperly, so consult your healthcare practitioner about other uses.

Peppermint

TIP *690*

FOR DIGESTIVE DISCOMFORT

Used as a remedy for indigestion for thousands of years, peppermint *(Mentha piperita)* relaxes the muscles of the digestive system and stimulates the stomach lining so that food spends less time churning within its walls. Commercial teas are widely available, but never ingest pure peppermint: It can cause cardiac arrhythmias.

Red Clover

TIP 691

BRONCHITIS BUSTER

For bronchitis, try an infusion of red clover *(Trifolium pratense)*;
it is both an anti-inflammatory agent and an expectorant that
helps remove excess mucus from the lungs. It also
helps purify the blood.

*Infusion: Steep 1 to 3 tsp of dried flower tops
in a cup of boiling water for 10 to 15 minutes, and
drink up to 3 cups a day.*

Red Raspberry

TIP 692

FOR PREGNANT WOMEN:
USE WITH CARE

Several herbal pregnancy formulas sold in the United States contain leaves of the red raspberry plant *(Rubus idaeus)*, because the
herb can help with the nausea and vomiting of morning sickness.
Red raspberry may also prevent miscarriage, strengthen
contractions during labor, reduce labor pain, and check
hemorrhaging. You should take it only under a
doctor's supervision during pregnancy.

Rose Hips

TIP 693

VITAMIN C FOR
COLDS AND FLU

The fruit of the genus *Rosa* contains high levels of vitamin C as well as flavonoids, which enhance the body's ability to use the vitamin that is a favorite for treating colds and flu. Since hips lose 45 to 90 percent of their C content through drying, try making your own jam from fresh fruit.

Jam: Collect the hips after the first frost, and do not use any from plants that have been sprayed with chemicals. Place them in a heavy stainless steel pan and simmer until tender, using 1 cup of water for each pound of rose hips. Rub through a fine sieve. Weigh the pulp and add an equal weight of heated sugar. Simmer the mixture until it is thick—and enjoy!

Sage

TIP 694

SAGE ADVICE

A mouthwash prepared with sage *(Salvia officinalis)* can help lick canker sores, bleeding gums, and sore throats by virtue of the plant's antiseptic oil as well as the astringent tannin that is concentrated in its leaves.

Mouthwash: Add 3 tsp leaves to 1 pint of water, bring to a boil, turn off the heat, and let the pan stand covered for 15 minutes. Gargle with the warm liquid three times a day.

Saw Palmetto

TIP 695

HERBAL HELP FOR PROSTATE PROBLEMS

Urination difficulties, bladder infections, and kidney problems in men over the age of 50 are often caused by a benign enlargement of the prostate gland. You may get help by taking gel capsules of saw palmetto *(Serenoa repens),* which seems to block production of the testosterone derivative that causes the condition. But first see a doctor to rule out prostate cancer, which has many of these same symptoms.

Skullcap

TIP 696

TONIC FOR THE NERVES

In case of tension headache, insomnia, or premenstrual symptoms aggravated by stress, try an over-the-counter tea containing the leaves and blue flowers of skullcap *(Scutellaria lateriflora),* which is reported to calm the nervous system. Don't overdo: Skullcap can cause drowsiness or confusion if taken in large amounts.

St.-John's-Wort

TIP 697

HOUSEHOLD HELP

Have on hand a commercial ointment of St.-John's-wort *(Hypericum perforatum)* for use the next time you get a minor cut, scrape, or burn. Herbalists have used it for centuries to heal such wounds.

Tea Tree Oil

TIP 698

SWEET-SMELLING
SKIN SOLUTION

A range of skin ailments, including athlete's foot, insect bites, cuts, and even teenage acne, respond to the nutmeg-scented oil of the tea tree (*Melaleuca* spp.), whose strong germicidal activity traces mainly to one ingredient, terpineol. You can purchase the oil to dab on affected skin; it's also a popular additive in health and beauty products such as soaps.

Turmeric

TIP 699

CURRY FAVOR

When arthritis pain flares, try this curry-flavored beverage made from *Curcuma longa*—commonly known as turmeric.

Tea: *Steep 1 tsp of the powdered root in 1 cup milk for 15 to 20 minutes; drink up to 3 cups a day.*

Uva Ursi

TIP 700

SELF-MADE ANTISEPTIC
FOR URINARY DISORDERS

Uva ursi (*Arctostaphylos uva-ursi*) contains arbutin, which is con- verted in the urinary tract into an antiseptic, making this herb an ideal treatment for mild bladder infections and urethritis. Try a commercial tea preparation or a tinc- ture—and don't panic if your urine turns dark green. This is a harmless side effect.

Valerian

TIP 701

HERBAL LULLABY

Perhaps the best cure available for insomnia, valerian *(Valeriana officinalis)* hastens the onset of sleep, causes none of the morning grogginess associated with drugs, does not interfere with REM sleep, and isn't habit forming.

Tea: Steep 2 tsp of dried, chopped valerian root in 1 cup of boiling water. Let it stand for eight to 12 hours and drink 1 cup just before bed.

Wild Yam

TIP 702

STAMP OUT CRAMPS

A capsule or two of wild yam *(Dioscorea villosa)* may be all you need to vanquish menstrual cramps. The extract, taken from the root of the plant, contains an alkaloid substance that relaxes the muscles of the entire abdominal region.

Yarrow

TIP 703

MULTIPLE LINES OF DEFENSE

Yarrow *(Achillea millefolium)* contains as many as 10 different compounds that help minor wounds heal; some are anti-inflammatory, some relieve pain, and some even help blood coagulate.

Compress: Steep 1 to 2 tsp of dried herb in 1 cup boiling water for 10 to 15 minutes, let cool, and apply to the wound with a cloth compress.

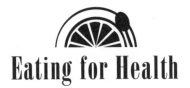

Eating for Health

NUTRITION,

VITAMINS,

MINERALS,

SUPPLEMENTS,

DIETARY

DOS AND DON'TS,

FOODS THAT HEAL

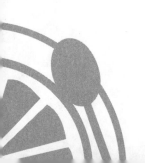

Eating for Health

TIP 704

THE SHAPE OF
GOOD NUTRITION

The current consensus on nutrition is represented by the food pyramid. The dietary foundation of the pyramid is grains (6 to 11 servings daily); next comes fruits and vegetables (6 to 9 servings); third, protein (2 to 3 servings of dairy and the same amount of meat, poultry, fish, eggs and nuts); last—and least—fats and sweets. A slice of bread is one serving of grain; a cup of milk constitutes one dairy serving; ½ cup of vegetables or a piece of fruit counts as one serving; one egg or 2 to 3 ounces of lean meat make up one protein serving.

TIP 705

LEAN AWAY FROM FAT

No more than 30 percent of your caloric intake should come from fat. (Some doctors recommend a limit of 25 or even 20 percent.) Saturated fat, which is found in artificially hardened vegetable oils like margarine, as well as in butter, cream, and meat, should be severely limited, especially among people with a genetic predisposition toward hardening of the arteries. If you already suffer from atherosclerosis and wish to try to reverse the condition through dietary modification, consult a doctor, especially if you are interested in going on the extremely low-fat diet (less than 10 percent) advocated by some practitioners.

TIP *706*

SENSIBLE CALORIES

More than half your caloric intake should come from whole
grains, vegetables, and fruits, which are rich in fiber and nutrients, and low in fat. Fruits are best consumed
whole, rather than as juices, which are high
in sugar and therefore calories. To rid fruits
and vegetables of pesticide residues, wash
them well in soapy water, rinse, and dry.

TIP *707*

SWEET MODERATION

Eat sugar and salt in moderation. Sugar (and this includes honey
and molasses) is high in calories and promotes tooth decay. Salt
may play a factor in high blood pressure; the fluid retention it
causes is also implicated in premenstrual syndrome (PMS), varicose veins, hemorrhoids, and the development of kidney stones.
Be aware that your salt shaker is probably not the main source of
salt in your diet. Prepared foods are generally very high in sugar
and sodium, so read labels carefully.

TIP *708*

VARY YOUR MENU

Don't eat the same meals every day, no matter how healthful they
are. To get all the nutrients you need, eat a variety of foods—if
not during a single day, at least over the course of a week.

TIP *709*

SUPPLEMENTAL INSURANCE

If your diet is ideal and you have no health problems, you probably don't need to take nutritional supplements. But if, like most people, you find it hard to follow the food pyramid guidelines, or are struggling with an ailment or injury, supplements can prove very helpful. But don't take megadoses (more than the recommended daily allowance) except under a doctor's supervision, since high levels of some vitamins can be toxic.

TIP *710*

RADICAL NOTIONS

Though the body needs a balance of nutrients, a group of vitamins and minerals called antioxidants is particularly important. This group—consisting of vitamins C, E, A, and the minerals selenium and chromium—can prevent unstable molecules known as free radicals from damaging cells and tissue. Because of this ability, the antioxidants are crucial in preventing cancer, preserving cardiovascular health, and optimizing immune system functioning. They can even help prevent cataracts and other degenerative eye diseases.

TIP *711*

THE POWER OF GARLIC

Garlic *(Allium sativum)* has a multitude of preventive and curative powers. The herb is thought to strengthen the cardiovascular system by reducing cholesterol and lowering blood pressure, fight infections by boosting immune system activity, and ease the irritation of colitis and other digestive problems. It can even even help get rid of warts. Ideally, it should be consumed raw, but if that's not palatable, add it to cooked GARLIC foods. Garlic capsules are another option.

TIP 712

SCALING BACK

Maintaining a normal weight is one of the most important things you can do to stay healthy. Unfortunately, it's also one of the most difficult. Drastically cutting calories—even if you can maintain such a Spartan regime—is likely to backfire, since your body may respond by lowering your fat-burning metabolism. To prevent this from happening, you need to maintain an adequate daily intake: at least 1,200 calories for a woman, 1,500 for a man. Kelp (*Fucus* spp.) tablets and dandelion *(Taraxacum officinale)* tea may help to boost your metabolism, but don't expect miracles. Aim for a slow, steady weight loss, or about three pounds a month. Unless you have a thyroid disorder or other medical problem, this should be achievable with a diet of vegetables, grains, and lean protein, along with regular, vigorous exercise.

DANDELION

TIP 713

START YOUR DAY RIGHT

Eat breakfast every day, even if you're not hungry when you wake up. Skipping the first meal is likely to make you overeat the wrong foods later in the day. Though you should have some fruit juice, you don't have to limit yourself to traditional morning fare. If you're in the mood for a piece of chicken—or any other protein that isn't high in fat—that's fine.

TIP 714

CRAVING CONTROL

Stress—especially the physical and emotional stress of dieting—can lead to binge eating. If you're hit by a sudden craving for a particular food, try waiting 20 minutes; often the desire will pass, especially if you go for a walk instead of staring into the refrigerator. If you must put something in your mouth right away, drink a glass of water, or have a small snack of something spicy.

TIP 715

THE SKINNY
ON BEING THIN

Yes, you can be too thin. If you're significantly below the norm on the standard weight charts but look healthy and feel energetic, don't worry. But if you look and feel weak, you should try to put on some pounds. You'll need to consume an extra 100-200 calories a day of lean meat, low-fat dairy products, and grain. Don't try to get the calories from candy or ice cream: It's muscle you want to gain, not fat. A program of weight training will help ensure that you stay in proportion.

TIP 716

ROUGHAGE MADE EASY

Nearly all Americans need to consume more fiber. A high-fiber diet can reduce the risk of colorectal cancer; it is also helpful in the prevention and treatment of various intestinal disorders, such as diverticulitis, irritable bowel syndrome, and ulcers. Fruits, vegetables, and grains are natural sources. But an easy way to ensure adequate fiber intake is with psyllium *(Plantago psyllium)*, available in drugstores as a powder that you mix with water.

TIP *717*

HYDROTHERAPY

A high-fiber diet can also help prevent constipation and the hemorrhoids that can result from straining to eliminate. In addition, many people find that the old folk remedy of a morning glass of warm water with the juice of a whole lemon in it can get the bowels moving. But with or without lemon, you should drink at least six glasses of water, juice, or herb tea a day.

TIP *718*

TUMMY TEAS

Although some people boast of their cast-iron stomachs, almost everyone experiences indigestion on occasion, generally after eating too much rich food. If indigestion is a frequent problem, try taking a bromelain capsule about a half hour before a meal. Teas that can be helpful after symptoms develop include chamomile *(Matricaria recutita)*, lemon balm *(Melissa officinalis)*, and peppermint *(Mentha piperita)*. And if you're a gum chewer, give your mouth a rest. It's usual for people who chew gum to simultaneously swallow air, which can cause digestive problems.

PEPPERMINT

TIP *719*

ROUTING GOUT

About half the people who develop gout have a hereditary predisposition toward the condition, which is caused by excessively high levels of uric acid in the blood. If there's a history of gout in your family, you may be able to prevent it from developing through changes in your diet. Eliminate red meat, particularly organ meats; shellfish; yeast; and alcohol. Treatment for gout involves avoiding sugar and drinking plenty of fluids—particularly cherry juice.

TIP 720

HAVE SOME
CABBAGE JUICE

Once prescribed for ulcer sufferers because of its purported soothing effect on the stomach, milk is now known to stimulate acid secretion, and should be avoided. A beverage to try—though it may take some getting used to—is cabbage juice, which increases the body's secretion of mucin, a substance that protects the stomach lining. Or you could try aloe vera juice, instead.

TIP 721

THE MILK MENACE

Milk and milk products can exacerbate a number of digestive disorders, including colitis and diverticulitis. After a bout of stomach flu or traveler's diarrhea, avoid dairy products other than yogurt for two weeks. Milk is also thought to increase mucus production, and is probably best avoided by people with respiratory problems, such as colds, hay fever, bronchitis, croup, sinusitis, asthma, and emphysema. Goat's milk causes less mucus production than cow's milk; soy milk is another alternative.

TIP 722

COOKOUT CAUTIONS

Barbecued foods—even healthy ones like fish—may pose a special risk. Researchers believe that the high heat leads to the formation of carcinogenic chemicals. To minimize the potential harm, trim fat from meat and poultry, don't baste it with oil or butter, don't cook it too close to the heat source, and take it off the grill before it is charred.

TIP 723

MEAT AND SKIN

If you suffer from eczema or psoriasis, try avoiding red meat and
see if the condition improves. Research suggests that an inability to metabolize fatty acids might be a culprit in these skin
disorders. Acidic fruits such as oranges and grapefruits can
also cause skin problems.

TIP 724

CHERRIES & COLLAGEN

Some nutritionists believe that people with arthritis should consume large quantities of cherries or other dark red berries.
The theory is that these fruits stimulate production of
collagen, which is essential to cartilage repair. Conversely, the alkaloids in tomatoes, potatoes, eggplants, and
peppers are thought to inhibit collagen formation.

TIP 725

GAS BUSTERS

There are a number of things you can do to prevent gas pains.
You should increase your fiber intake, slowly, since high-fiber
foods can temporarily make gas worse. Meals should be smaller,
with fewer different food items on the plate. As for that notori-
ous gas producer, beans, there are a few ways to make them
more digestible. You should soak dry beans overnight, and skim
the foam from them when you cook them. But if this doesn't
work, and you don't get any relief by switching to less gaseous
legumes, try a widely available drugstore product that contains
an enzyme that breaks down the indigestible sugars in beans.
Other foods that can cause problems are alcohol, carbonated
beverages, cheese, and soy sauce.

TIP 726

STONE BARRIERS

People prone to kidney stones should also avoid foods that raise uric acid levels, and should probably reduce their consumption of chocolate, grapes, spinach, asparagus, and green peppers, all of which contain calcium oxalate. Cutting down on salt and drinking large quantities of fluids is also recommended. But check with your doctor to find out exactly what dietary measures are indicated.

TIP 727

SALTED HEARING?

If your hearing is failing, you might want to try cutting back on dietary salt; excess sodium consumption can cause fluid retention in the ear, exacerbating hearing problems. There is also evidence that beta carotene supplements (5,000 to 10,000 IU a day) can be helpful, particularly if the hearing loss is accompanied by the ringing in the ears known as tinnitus.

TIP 728

FAST RELIEF
FROM ALLERGIES

Fasting may help your body fight allergies. Some practitioners believe that consuming only juice or water releases a hormone that enhances immune system activity. Fasting also may reduce stress on the body's defense system by saving the energy that would otherwise go to processing food allergens. Fasting should be done under the supervision of a doctor or nutritionist.

TIP *729*

A HONEY OF A
HAY FEVER REMEDY

People who suffer from hay fever can be helped by consuming honey, according to some researchers. Two months before the season starts, begin eating 2 tsp daily of raw honey that comes from a nearby hive. And since vitamin C and bioflavonoids act as natural antihistamines, you should increase your citrus intake or take 500 mg of the vitamin three times daily.

TIP *730*

THOSE
CANTANKEROUS SORES

If you have a tendency to develop canker sores, try avoiding caffeine, decaffeinated beverages, spices, and citrus fruits, which may irritate your mouth. Taking supplements of vitamins C and B complex, as well as folic acid, iron, and zinc, may also be helpful, as is eating yogurt every day. The same dietary restrictions apply if you have a cold sore; the nutritional treatment for frequent cold sores is lysine supplementation, 200 mg a day.

TIP *731*

THE JAWBONE'S
CONNECTED TO THE MENU

To avoid putting strain on jaw muscles and joints, people who
suffer the facial pain and recurrent headaches of TMJ
(temporomandibular joint) syndrome should avoid
difficult-to-chew foods like carrots, apples, steak,
and bagels, as well as foods that stimulate the adrenal
glands, such as white sugar, coffee, caffeine, and decaffeinated beverages. During TMJ flare-ups, going on a liquid diet
for a day or two can be helpful.

TIP *732*

EATING FOR BETTER BREATH

If you've got bad breath in spite of good dental hygiene, chances
are that your bad breath is being caused by bad digestion. Improving your diet, by eating more whole grains, fresh fruit
(especially saliva-stimulating oranges and grapefruits),
and raw vegetables, will improve your digestion and help
eliminate mouth odor. Chewing fresh parsley or peppermint leaves can be a quick fix. And don't skip breakfast,
unless you want your morning breath to last till lunch.

TIP *733*

DRINKING OFF
A HANGOVER

It was a great party, but now you're paying for it with a morning-
after hangover. Forget about the hair-of-the-dog; instead, drink
diluted fruit juices to help burn off the alcohol. Bouillon will
restore your body's electrolyte balance. If nausea is a problem,
munch on crackers and honey.

TIP 734

SOME CHILLING NEWS
ABOUT HOT TODDIES

Though a hot toddy might seem like just the thing if you're suffering from cold hands and feet, if your icy appendages are caused by circulatory problems, lay off the booze. Although drinking will temporarily warm you up, alcohol ultimately makes it more difficult to maintain body temperature and can even promote hypothermia.

TIP 735

SPORTS NUTRITION

Don't work out for at least two to three hours after a heavy meal. Instead, have a piece of fruit or other high-carbohydrate snack an hour before exercising; 15 minutes before, drink a large glass of water. Avoid sugar and caffeine, which can tighten muscles, increasing the risk of injury.

TIP 736

SWEAT EQUITY

Excessive sweating may be linked to a zinc deficiency; taking 30 to 60 mg. of zinc daily may help solve the problem. To treat body odor that is not controlled by frequent washing with antibacterial agents and the use of an antiperspirant, try taking chlorophyll, a natural plant product available in tablet form.

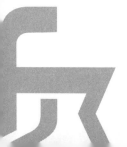

Exercising for Health

SIMPLE,

PRACTICAL

ROUTINES FOR

DAILY FITNESS—PLUS

VALUABLE TIPS

ON GETTING

THE MOST FROM

YOUR WORKOUT

_____

Exercising for Health

TIP *737*

FOCUS ON FOUR

For optimal fitness, combine:
1. aerobic exercise for your heart and circulatory system;
2. weight training for strong muscles and bones;
3. flexibility exercises for supple joints; and
4. a healthy diet to keep your body fat percentage at ideal levels.

TIP *738*

A DOCTOR'S OKAY

Check with your doctor before starting an exercise program if you've been sedentary, are taking medications, are 65 or older, or have health problems such as chest pains or high blood pressure.

TIP *739*

SETTING GOALS

Set specific, achievable, short-term goals that balance challenge with reality. If you're just starting to swim laps, for instance, don't target the English Channel sometime in the next 10 years. Do target 20 laps in the next month.

TIP *740*

THINK "4-20-60" FOR FITNESS

Exercise four times a week, for at least 20 minutes a session, at no less than 60 percent of your maximal heart rate. Four times is significantly better than three.

TIP 741

SUSTAINING VARIETY

Mix and match different workouts to keep your interest level high. If you're a jogger, for instance, consider swimming, riding a bike, or playing tennis once a week. Cross-training is one of the most effective ways to keep from quitting an exercise program.

TIP 742

TAKE IT SLOWER—LONGER

Exercise at a moderate intensity level for a relatively longer period. The opposite approach—high intensity for a shorter time—will give you the same cardiovascular benefits, but it's also more likely to lead to injuries, which could sideline you completely.

TIP 743

EXERCISE IS CUMULATIVE

If you can't always schedule a single block of time for exercise, try accumulating 30 minutes or more piecemeal over the course of your day. A 15-minute walk, 10 minutes spent weeding the garden, a five-minute wrestling match with your kids, and five one-minute stair climbs can do you a world of good.

TIP *744*

STEPS TOWARD HEALTH

Try walking 30 minutes a day, most days of the week. Walking is a terrific form of exercise that requires no expensive gear, targets the body's largest muscle groups, puts little strain on joints, and can be done alone or with companions almost anywhere. If you hate "exercise," try thinking of it less as something to be done at the gym, and more like just a natural part of your day. Walk on short errands, take the stairs instead of the elevator, and don't cruise the parking lot for the closest space to the mall.

TIP *745*

THE RACE IS NOT ALWAYS TO THE SWIFT

Think you can't walk fast enough to do yourself any good? Think again. Researchers have found that slow-walking a given distance produces virtually the same cardiovascular benefits as fast-walking the same course.

TIP *746*

EXERCISE IN THE ZONE

To become aerobically fit, keep your heart beating within a "target zone" of 60 to 85 percent of its age-predicted maximum while you train. Calculate this zone by subtracting your age from 220, then multiplying the result by 60 percent for the low end of the range, then by 85 percent for the upper end. If you're a serious athlete, calculate a more precise "target zone" by subtracting both your age and your resting heart rate from 220, multiplying this result by 50 and 90 percent respectively, then adding back your resting heart rate.

WARMING UP, COOLING DOWN

To prevent injuries and get the most from your aerobic workout, begin with a five- to 10-minute warmup period of stretching and low-intensity exercise. End your workout with a similar cooldown period. Go with the feel, to decide if a given stretching exercise is good for you. You'll feel a healthy stretch in your muscles—a not-so-healthy one in your joints.

TIP 748

A BETTER SIT-UP

The best way to exercise your abs is by doing a slow curl up, only to the point where your midback is off the floor. Remember to keep your knees bent. This modified sit-up works better—and with less risk of lower-back strain—than the full, straight-legged sit-ups you were probably taught in grade school.

TIP 749

DON'T WAIT TO EXHALE

Whenever lifting weights or performing strengthening calisthenics like pushups, remember to exhale during exertion and inhale as you return to the starting position.

TIP 750

HOMEMADE WEIGHTS

Use plastic water jugs as light weights for exercise. Add 2 cups of water for each pound; a gallon weighs nearly eight pounds.

TIP 751

ONCE IS ENOUGH

When strength-training, do a single set of repetitions for each exercise. In the past, trainers recommended two or even three sets, but researchers have recently found that one set increases strength and muscle density just as effectively as two or more.

TIP 752

THE PROPER TOE TOUCH

Sit, don't stand, when touching your toes. The seated toe touch, with your legs outstretched and knees unlocked, will let you safely stretch your hamstrings without causing strain on your lower back the way yesteryear's standing toe touch can.

TIP 753

THE DOG AND CAT

Try two great yoga stretches for your back and hips.

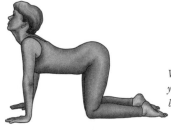

Dog
While on your hands and knees, inhale as you dip your back, bringing your head and buttocks up. Exhale as you return your back to the horizontal.

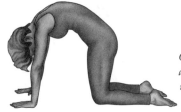

Cat
On your hands and knees, exhale as you arch your back, stretching your shoulder, neck, and back muscles. Inhale and bring your back to the horizontal.

TIP *754*

BODY FAT GUIDELINES

Eating right and exercising your whole body will help you reduce fat levels. Unfortunately, you can't spot-reduce fat, from saddle-bags to cellulite, by targeting a particular body area for exercise. Optimal body fat percentages are 18 percent or less for men and 25 percent or less for women. You can have your body fat composition calculated at a local gym.

TIP *755*

BODY MASS INDEX

Combine diet and exercise to keep your body mass index (BMI) between 19 and 25. To calculate your own score:

1. Take your weight in pounds and divide it by 2.2.
2. Take your height in inches, divide it by 39.4, then multiply this result by itself.
3. Finally, divide step 1 by step 2.

TIP *756*

FAT AND ULTRA SPORTS

If you plan to compete in a race longer than 10K, boost dietary fat to 30 to 45 percent of total calories in the weeks before the race. A study found that athletes who ate this diet increased their overall endurance by 14 percent and were much less prone to experiencing exercise-induced muscle fatigue.

TIP *757*

NO GAIN FROM PAIN

Listen to your body's early-warning signals, and don't push yourself to play through pain. Overexertion can cause painful swelling of muscles and joints as well as leave you chronically tired.

TIP *758*

RECIPE FOR A PAINFREE BACK

Strengthen your abdominal muscles and stretch your hamstrings as a regular part of your fitness routine. This simple exercise combination will significantly decrease your risk of lower-back pain.

TIP *759*

THE IMPACT OF IMPACT

To help avoid injuries, alternate high-impact sports like running or basketball with more joint-friendly low-impact sports like hiking, rowing, bike riding, swimming, or cross-country skiing.

TIP *760*

PAIN RELIEF

To treat muscle aches and joint pains stemming from overexertion, try anti-inflammatory drugs like aspirin or ibuprofen, heat rubs or massage with an aspirin-containing cream, or the homeopathic remedy *Arnica*.

TIP 761

TENNIS ELBOW

Combat the painful inflammation known as tennis elbow with rest, anti-inflammatory drugs like aspirin, and exercises to stretch and strengthen elbow muscles. Avoid bracing your arm with a band worn below the elbow, a popular presumed remedy that does more harm than good.

TIP 762

SEEK ACUPUNCTURE TREATMENT

Acupuncture has an estimated 60 to 70 percent success rate when used on tennis elbow patients—a record that has helped it gain acceptance even in more conservative medical circles. There are a number of acupuncture points that might prove beneficial, so be sure to seek out an acupuncturist who is experienced in treating this or similar types of conditions.

TIP 763

DROWN OUT MUSCLE CRAMPS

If you get cramps while exercising or doing other activities that cause you to sweat, you are probably dehydrated. Physical overexertion depletes the body's fluids and minerals, particularly potassium and sodium, which can lead to cramping. To avoid cramps, be sure to drink 6 to 8 cups of water every day. And take frequent water breaks during long athletic practices or events. If you suspect that a mineral imbalance is contributing to your cramping, try a carbohydrate-electrolyte sports drink. Choose one that is low in sugar; in an overheated body, sugar can bring on stomach cramps. Never take salt tablets; they can actually cause you to lose more minerals, sometimes to dangerously low levels.

TIP *764*

EYE GUARDS

If you spend much time exercising in the sun, make sure to protect your eyes with sunglasses rated for broad-spectrum UV protection. In general, gray lenses block UV rays more effectively than brown or green ones.

TIP *765*

FORGIVING SURFACES
BEST FOR SHIN SPLINTS

Joggers prone to the common affliction of the lower leg known as shin splints should invest in a good pair of running shoes and be sure to exercise on forgiving surfaces: Wood chips, earth tracks, and other resilient surfaces are much better choices than concrete pavement.

TIP *766*

BEATING BLISTERS

Protect your feet from blisters by breaking in new running shoes gradually and applying petroleum jelly or calendula ointment and a bandage to blister-prone areas. Acrylic-fiber athletic socks with heels (not tube socks) are best because of their low friction.

TIP *767*

ALTERNATIVE HEALING

Apply a poultice of gardenia *(Gardenia jasminoides)*, flour, and wine to reduce swelling and promote healing of minor strains or sprains. Massaging with safflower flower *(Carthamus tinctorius)* can also help speed recovery.

TIP 768

SUPPLEMENTARY HEALING

To foster your body's ability to heal minor sports injuries, take 1,000 mg of vitamin C, 10,000 IU of beta carotene, 60 mg of zinc, and 400 IU of vitamin E daily.

TIP 769

COLD RELIEF

During cold season, follow regular, moderate exercise with a sauna twice a week. Regular exercise appears to strengthen the immune system, and the heat from a sauna may keep cold viruses from reproducing. Just make sure to drink plenty of water.

TIP 770

WHEN HEAT STRIKES

If you feel faint, nauseated, headachy, or dizzy during exercise on a hot day, stop your workout and drink water, seek shade or air-conditioning, and apply cold compresses to cool your body. If you stop sweating during exercise, take these actions immediately, then seek medical help. No sweat is a symptom of heat stroke, which can be deadly.

TIP 771

POUR ON THE WATER

Remember to drink a cup of water 15 to 30 minutes before exercising. If the weather is hot or your exercise intensity is high, make sure to stop and replenish fluids every 15 to 20 minutes. And drink water when you're done exercising as well.

TIP 772

THE SEXUAL SOLUTION

Researchers have found that sexual intercourse before a major competition does not hinder athletic performance—in fact, it may even enhance performance by reducing precompetition anxiety.

TIP 773

SWIMMING WITH ASTHMA

If you suffer from asthma, try swimming. Not only will you get a great aerobic workout, but the increased humidity can help ease breathing. Just make sure to keep your medication poolside—and be ready to stop if you find chlorine bothersome.

TIP 774

HEALTHY LOOP

Don't let rain, snow, or oppressive heat stop you from your daily walk. Just find a shopping mall and take a hike indoors.

TIP 775

TRAFFIC CONGESTION

Never jog on streets with heavy traffic. Besides the obvious increased danger of accidents, you'll inhale unhealthy levels of carbon monoxide and other pollutants.

TIP 776

EXERCISE YOUR MIND

Exercise aerobically if you want to improve your mind. Sedentary individuals who take up regular aerobic exercise score significant gains in memory, mental flexibility, response time, and other cognitive measures.

TIP 777

PEER SUPPORT

Join a team or exercise with a buddy. Social reinforcement and gentle peer pressure make workouts fun—and keep you going on days you're tempted to skip.

TIP 778

LOVING EXERCISE

Improve your sex life with vigorous exercise—but you have to sweat to achieve this. A study of reformed couch potatoes found that spirited aerobic exercise led to a jump in sexual desire and intercourse. A second test group walked for an hour four times a week; they got healthier but didn't enjoy the sexual boost.

TIP 779

AFTER BURN

Use exercise to burn more calories at rest. Researchers have discovered that people who exercise regularly continue to burn excess calories for several hours after finishing a workout.

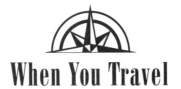

When You Travel

Your passport

to health on

the road—from

vital health info

about traveling

abroad to

stay-well tips for

business trips

———————

When You Travel

TIP 780

DON'T LEAVE HOME WITHOUT IT

Your health insurance might end at the border. Find out whether your coverage extends to overseas trips; if it doesn't, you can buy a traveler's policy from your tour group or credit card company.

TIP 781

BOOSTERISM

Check with the health department to see what immunizations you'll need if you're planning a trip to the developing world. And wherever you're heading, make sure your tetanus protection is up to date: You need a booster shot every 10 years.

TIP 782

TRAVELING FOR TWO

Pregnant women should find out when—and if—it's okay to travel. In general, the second trimester is the safest.

TIP 783

DENTAL INSURANCE

If you're due (or overdue) to see your dentist, stop procrastinating. Schedule a checkup, allowing enough time for any work that might be necessary.

TIP *784*

TROPICAL ADVICE

If you're heading into malaria country—which includes most
tropical and subtropical zones—let your doctor
know well in advance. You'll probably need to
begin an antimalaria regime, and the drugs
take several weeks to become effective. For additional protection, use mosquito repellents and
wear long pants and sleeves.

TIP *785*

A PRESCRIPTION FOR YOUR HEALTH

Make sure you don't run out of any essential medication. Get
enough from your pharmacist to last your whole trip, and pack it
in your carry-on, not in luggage you'll be checking. To avoid
problems with customs, keep drugs in their original containers.

TIP *786*

MISHAPS WILL HAPPEN

Take along a basic first-aid kit: alcohol, bandages, aspirin,
antacids, cough syrup.

TIP 787

THE VISION THING

You can't enjoy the sights unless you can see them. If broken glasses would ruin your trip, take along an extra pair.

TIP 788

DON'T LEAVE YOUR PAST BEHIND

If you have a serious health problem, bring a copy of your medical records. And also be sure you include information about any medications you may be allergic to.

TIP 789

BAGGAGE CHECK

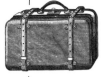

Try not to pack more than you can comfortably carry. If that's not possible, invest in a wheeled luggage rack, to take a load off your back and shoulders.

TIP 790

STEP SMART

Forget about making a footwear fashion statement. Your traveling wardrobe should include two pairs of broken-in walking shoes, and a generous supply of athletic socks.

TIP 791

KEEP A CLEAR HEAD

Avoid flying if you have an ear or sinus infection, or a severe head cold. With a mild cold, clear your nasal passages—and stave off ear problems—by using a long-lasting decongestant spray.

TIP 792

WHEN FLYING WITH A COLD

If you take a plane trip with a stuffy nose you may encounter an extremely painful condition known as aerotitis medica, or barotrauma—a pushing in of the eardrum caused by the sudden increase in air pressure in the plane's cabin as the plane descends. Your best bet is not to fly with a cold or sinus infection. But if you must, be sure to take the following preventive steps:

- Use a nasal decongestant or antihistamine an hour before takeoff and again an hour before landing.
- Suck on candy or chew gum to promote swallowing and help unblock the Eustachian tubes.
- To unblock your ear passages during your flight, take a deep breath through your mouth, hold your nose, and then blow out gently while keeping your mouth closed.
- Take the homeopathic remedy *Kali bichromicum* in 6c or 30c potency at half-hour intervals during your flight, starting a half-hour before boarding your plane.

TIP 793

MENU PLANNING

On a flight where food will be served, let the airline know at least a day ahead if you're on a restricted diet. The airline can generally supply a low-sodium, low-cholesterol, diabetic, or other special meal.

TIP 794

DON'T FLY DRY

While you're airborne, drink plenty of water and juice. Avoid alcohol and caffeinated beverages, both of which stimulate your kidneys to produce more urine and thus dehydrate you faster.

TIP 795

PREPARE FOR THE WORST

It's easier to prevent motion sickness than to treat it. An over-the-counter medication like the brand-name drug Dramamine, taken a half hour before a trip, can head off minor problems. If you need a stronger drug, your doctor can prescribe a scopolamine ear patch. For an alternative, try the homeopathic remedy *Nux vomica*. Take it at 30c strength as the plane takes off, and then as needed.

TIP 796

SITTING PRETTY

For a smoother ride, ask the airline for a seat over the wings. On a ship, book a midsection cabin. On a train or bus, always choose a seat facing forward.

TIP 797

TANK UP BEFORE
YOU HIT THE ROAD

Don't go away hungry; an empty stomach is more easily upset than a full one. Eat a small, low-fat meal shortly before your departure, and have a snack—crackers are a safe bet—every couple of hours during a long trip.

TIP 798

WRIST MANAGEMENT

Acupressure wristbands, available at many pharmacies and sporting-goods stores, can quell queasiness. You can also use your thumb to stimulate the pressure points on the inside of your wrists.

Lung 7
On the thumb side of the inner forearm, measure two finger widths above the crease in the wrist. Apply steady, firm pressure to the point site with your thumb, then repeat on the other arm.

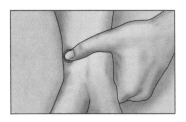

TIP 799

KEEP A COOL HEAD

An ice bag, held against the base of the skull for 15 minutes, can help relieve motion sickness.

TIP *800*

READING?
KEEP YOUR NOSE IN THE BOOK

People susceptible to motion sickness shouldn't read during trips —in fact, they should try to keep their eyes closed. But if you're on a business trip and must look over some papers, turn your back to the window, slouch in your seat, and hold the documents at eye level.

TIP *801*

CLOCK YOURSELF

Three days before a cross-country or transoceanic flight, adjust your sleep schedule. If it's at all possible and practical, go to bed—and wake up—according to the clock in the time zone you'll be heading into.

TIP *802*

THE EVENING ADVANTAGE

To minimize jet lag, try to arrange your trip so that you'll arrive in the early evening. In other words, take an early flight when traveling east, a late one when heading west.

TIP *803*

GOOD MORNING, SUNSHINE

Don't nap during the day you arrive, or sleep late the next morning. Get up at your usual hour (destination time), and get out into the sun. Exposure to daylight will reset your internal clock.

TIP *804*

EXERCISE CAUTION

Exercise will help you feel better after a long flight. But if you're going to be arriving late at night, skip the workout; it will make it harder to fall asleep and get your internal clock reset.

TIP *805*

MEAT AND POTATOES

If your first meal in a new time zone is breakfast or lunch, consume plenty of protein. The evening meal should be heavy on carbohydrates.

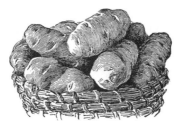

TIP *806*

TO THE RESCUE

The Bach flower essence remedy known as Rescue Remedy can help fight jet lag by regulating body rhythms and alleviating stress. Take it when you take off, then every hour.

TIP *807*

AND NOT A DROP TO DRINK

Even in the developed world, it can take a while for your intestinal system to adjust to the water. But in the developing world, tap water can make you seriously ill—so don't drink it, cook with it, or brush your teeth with it. (The same goes for water from a spring or stream.) To avoid water-borne illnesses:

- Pack an immersion coil, and boil water for at least 10 minutes.
- Use water-purifying tablets, available at drugstores and from outdoor outfitters.
- If you buy bottled water, make sure the seal is unbroken.
- Avoid ice cubes, unless they're made with water you've treated yourself.

TIP *808*

GET INTO COOL WATER

Walking more than you're used to can leave your feet swollen and sore. Soak away the pain in a basin of cool water mixed with Epsom salts.

TIP *809*

ALIMENTARY PRECAUTIONS

The more exotic your destination, the more you'll have to watch
what you eat as well as what you drink.

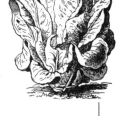

- Avoid lettuce and other raw vegetables.
- Stay away from fruit, unless you can peel
  it yourself.
- Don't eat raw or undercooked meat or fish.
  Raw seafood is particularly risky.
- Beware: Unpasteurized milk and cheeses are
  another potential hazard.

TIP *810*

ONE A DAY WHEN YOU'RE AWAY

If you'll be spending a substantial amount of time in a country
where you may find it hard to eat a balanced diet, bring along a
supply of multivitamins. One acidophilus capsule taken two times
a day will keep your balance of good bacteria right.

TIP *811*

GET IN THE PINK

Some travelers swear that the well-known brand name medication
Pepto-Bismol, begun before a trip and continued after you're
back home, can help prevent intestinal and digestive problems
associated with traveling. Check with your doctor about dosages.

TIP *812*

BLOCKING THE RUNS

Since diarrhea is the body's way of ridding itself of toxins, some experts recommend that you let it run its course. But if you're unable to wait it out, the medicine loperamide, available in prescription and nonprescription doses in the United States, is a quick fix.

TIP *813*

ACTIVATE SOME CHARCOAL

Charcoal can also help with watery bowel movements. Take two capsules with a glass of water after each episode of the runs.

TIP *814*

DRUGSTORE DANGERS

Stay away from antidiarrheal medicines available over the counter in foreign countries: The FDA has found many of them to be unsafe. Instead, if you're troubled by diarrhea, bring along any of the following homeopathic remedies: *Arsenicum, Nux vomica, Phosphorus.*

TIP *815*

FORCE FLUIDS

If you develop diarrhea, you'll need to rehydrate yourself. Drink plenty of bottled juices and caffeine-free soft drinks. If it is available, a sports drink like Gatorade can help replace lost minerals. Or you can add a teaspoon of sugar and a pinch of salt to a glass of juice.

TIP *816*

EASE BACK INTO SOLID FOODS

Stay on a liquid diet until the diarrhea is over. When you begin eating again, start out with easy-to-digest foods like rice, crackers, bananas, and applesauce.

TIP *817*

DIPLOMATIC ASSISTANCE

Should you need medical attention while you are overseas, contact the American Embassy; it can generally provide you with a list of English-speaking doctors. The Red Cross is another resource.

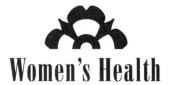

Women's Health

TIPS FOR

THE SPECIAL

HEALTH CONCERNS

OF WOMEN

OF ALL AGES—

INCLUDING

NATURAL ALTERNATIVE

TREATMENTS AND

PREVENTION

———————

Women's Health

TIP *818*

VITAMIN E FOR BREAST PAIN

For breast pain not caused by cancer, many doctors recommend vitamin E supplements in daily doses of 600 to 800 IU.

TIP *819*

WHEN NOT TO USE TAMPONS

If you have endometriosis, a condition in which pieces of the lining of the uterus (endometrium) migrate out of the uterus and begin to grow on other organs and tissues within the abdomen, then you may wish to avoid using tampons altogether. Some health practitioners believe that tampons encourage menstrual flow to back up—one theory for the cause of endometriosis.

TIP *820*

PHYTOS FIGHT
HOT FLASHES, TOO

Eating soybeans and other foods high in phytoestrogens (plant estrogens) may help alleviate the hot flashes associated with menopause. This may help explain why very few women in Japan, where soybeans are a staple food, report difficulty with hot flashes. Wheat, olives, plums, carrots, apples, yams, and coconuts are among the other foods that contain phytoestrogens.

TIP *821*

AVOID FLASH FOODS

If you suffer from hot flashes, cut back on foods that have been implicated as possible triggers of hot flashes. These include: caffeinated and decaffeinated coffees, teas and colas; chocolate; alcohol; and excessively spicy, salty, or sugary foods. Some women also report that hot soups and drinks or very large meals can set off a hot flash.

TIP *822*

POINT OF RELIEF

To help relieve the discomfort of menstrual cramping, try applying pressure to the acupressure point known as Liver 3.

Liver 3
Place your index fingers next to the large knuckle of each big toe, then press into the groove on top of the foot between the big toe and the second toe.

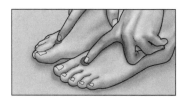

TIP *823*

A FEMALE TONIC

Since ancient times, herbalists have used the berries of the chaste tree *(Vitex agnus-castus)*, sometimes known as chasteberries, to treat various female conditions. Today, chasteberries are often prescribed for menstrual irregularity, premenstrual syndrome and menopausal symptoms. The berries are also said to help the body readjust after withdrawal from long-term use of birth-control pills and to promote lactation. For optimal benefit, the herb should be taken for six months or longer.

CHASTE TREE

Tea: *Pour 1 cup boiling water onto 1 tsp ripe berries and let them infuse for 10 to 15 minutes; drink three times a day.*

TIP *824*

NO SEX. PERIOD.

If you have a history of pelvic infections or have several sexual partners, avoid intercourse during your menstrual period. The cervix—the opening to the uterus—widens during menstruation to allow blood and uterine tissue to flow out. This widening also permits bacteria from contaminated semen to enter the normally sterile uterus.

TIP *825*

NUX FOR NAUSEA

Two frequently recommended homeopathic remedies for morning sickness are the following:

- ***Nux vomica*** (30c) for intense nausea with irritability.
- ***Tabacum*** (30c) for persistent queasiness with a sense of hopelessness.

Follow label directions or consult a homeopathic physician.

TIP *826*

WATCH WHAT
(AND WHEN) YOU EAT

If you suffer from premenstrual syndrome (PMS), try reducing your intake of caffeine, sugar, salt, dairy products, and white flour, which studies have shown can sometimes aggravate PMS symptoms. Eating six or more small meals throughout the day rather than three large ones can also reduce PMS symptoms, perhaps by keeping insulin levels more constant.

TIP *827*

TAKE AN HERBAL BATH

By easing tension and stress, a long, warm bath can help relieve some of the symptoms associated with PMS. To the bathwater add several drops of lavender *(Lavandula officinalis)*, chamomile *(Matricaria recutita)*, parsley *(Petroselinum crispum)*, or juniper *(Juniperus communis)* oil. To relieve premenstrual breast tenderness, try adding 6 to 8 drops of geranium *(Pelargonium odoratissimum)* oil to the water.

PARSLEY

TIP *828*

FOR FAST RELIEF

For immediate relief from breast pain and swelling during your menstrual cycle, apply a warm castor-oil pack to your breast. Saturate a flannel cloth with high-grade castor oil, put it over your breast, and cover it with plastic wrap and a towel; apply heat to the pack using a heating pad or hot-water bottle, and leave it on for 20 to 30 minutes.

TIP *829*

SLICE FAT FROM YOUR FOODS

Some studies suggest that limiting dietary fat—especially saturated fat—may help shrink or eliminate benign breast lumps. Other studies have shown a link between high-fat diets and breast cancer. Although these connections have not been definitely proven, you should cut back on dietary fat for another, well-accepted reason: A low-fat diet reduces your risk of heart disease, the leading cause of premature death in women.

TIP *830*

STRETCH AFTER SURGERY

To help restore your mobility and reduce muscle stiffness after breast surgery, try this simple yoga exercise, known as Climbing the Wall.

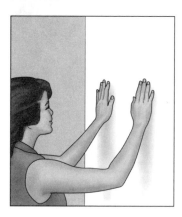

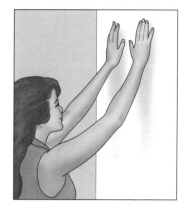

Stand approximately a foot from a wall with your feet slightly apart. Place both hands on the wall.

Slowly slide your hands up the wall as far as you can, but stop immediately if you feel any pain. Repeat five times a day, with the goal of raising both arms above your head.

TIP *831*

A GOLDEN HERB

Goldenseal *(Hydrastis canadensis)* douches are recommended for cervicitis and cervical erosion, two common inflammatory conditions of the cervix.

Douche: Pour 1 cup boiling water over 1 tbsp goldenseal. Steep for 15 minutes, then strain and use warm. Pour into a douche container and use as directed on the container package. Repeat every day until symptoms are gone.

GOLDENSEAL

TIP *832*

IMMEDIATE PAIN RELIEF

To help relieve the cramping pain associated with endometriosis, try applying pressure to the acupressure point known as Spleen 6.

Spleen 6
Measure four finger widths up from the top of the right inside anklebone. With your thumb, press near the edge of the shinbone. Repeat on the other leg. (Do not apply pressure to this point if you are pregnant.)

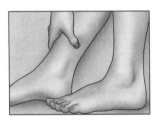

TIP *833*

PUT THE SQUEEZE ON STRESS INCONTINENCE

If you suffer from stress incontinence—an involuntary loss of urine while coughing, sneezing, laughing, exercising, or otherwise moving in a way that puts sudden pressure on the bladder—you may benefit from doing Kegel exercises, which strengthen the pelvic floor muscles that support the uterus and bladder.

The exercises are quite simple: Slowly contract your pelvic floor muscles. Hold for up to 10 seconds and repeat several times. You can do the exercises while standing, sitting, or lying down. Do not do Kegels while urinating, as the practice may push urine back up to the kidneys, raising the risk of infection.

TIP *834*

VITAMIN E FOR HOT FLASHES

Many women report that taking 400 to 800 IU of vitamin E daily helps minimize the frequency and intensity of their hot flashes during menopause. Vitamin E has also been linked to a reduced risk of cardiovascular disease.

TIP *835*

HEALTH FLASH FROM CHINA

To lessen the intensity of hot flashes and other symptoms of menopause, you may want to try the Chinese herbs dong quai *(Angelica sinensis)* and Asian ginseng *(Panax ginseng)*. Both contain natural plant estrogens, or phytoestrogens, and have been reported to help relieve hot flashes. Because these herbs can be toxic at some dosages, you should consult an experienced herbalist before using them.

TIP *836*

NATURAL LUBRICANTS

Several estrogenic herbal creams are available to help relieve the vaginal dryness and dry skin that sometimes accompany menopause. Consult your healthcare practitioner or an herbalist for a recommendation. Some couples also report breaking open capsules of vitamin E and massaging them on as a natural lubricant for postmenopausal lovemaking.

TIP *837*

KEEP A HOT-FLASH JOURNAL

Keep a written record of your hot flashes. Write down when the flash occurs, its intensity (on a scale of 1 to 5), and what precipitated it. Look for patterns in your flashes. Such knowledge will help you predict and manage your flashes better.

TIP *838*

TRY ACUPUNCTURE

In one small Swedish study, women who received acupuncture treatment for their menopausal symptoms reported a 50 percent drop in the frequency of their hot flashes. If you decide to try acupuncture, be sure to seek out an experienced practitioner.

TIP *839*

A BARK FOR CRAMPS

The aptly named cramp bark *(Viburnum opulus)* is a traditional herbal remedy for relieving the pain of menstrual cramps. Teas made from ginger *(Zingiber officinale)*, bilberry *(Vaccinium myrtillus)*, dong quai *(Angelica sinensis)*, and feverfew *(Chrysanthemum parthenium)* can also help relax uterine muscles and relieve menstrual cramping.

GINGER   *Cramp bark tea: Simmer 2 tsp of the dried bark in 1 cup of water for 15 minutes; drink three times a day.*

TIP *840*

CUT OUT CAFFEINE

Caffeine can aggravate menstrual cramping and menopausal hot flashes. If you suffer regularly from either of these conditions, you may want to wean yourself off caffeine. Remember: Caffeine is found not only in coffee, but also in chocolate, black and green tea, and cola and many other soft drinks.

TIP *841*

MASSAGE AWAY CRAMPS

To help relieve the pain of menstrual cramps, massage your lower abdomen, back, and legs with oil or lotion containing chamomile *(Matricaria recutita)*. Evening primrose oil *(Oenothera biennis)* can also be rubbed over painful areas to bring relief. (Do not use evening primrose oil, however, if there is a chance you may be pregnant.)

CHAMOMILE

TIP *842*

TAKE A WALK

Although you may feel like crawling into bed when you have menstrual cramps, getting up and walking may be a much better idea. Walking improves circulation to the pelvic organs and reduces muscle tension. So when the cramps hit, you should hit the pavement for a long stroll at a comfortable, relaxed pace.

TIP *843*

YOGA RELIEF

The Downward Dog yoga pose helps release pelvic tension and thus relieve menstrual cramping.

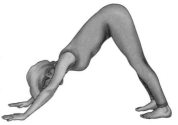

Downward Dog
Get on your hands and knees. Inhale and raise your pelvis to form an inverted V, with knees slightly bent. Press your palms and heels against the floor as you breathe deeply. Hold for 20 to 30 seconds. Exhale as you return to the starting position.

TIP *844*

YARROW TO SLOW THE FLOW

To help control heavy menstrual bleeding, try yarrow *(Achillea millefolium)* tea. Another remedy is a tincture made of equal parts life root *(Senecio aureus)*, shepherd's purse *(Capsella bursa-pastoris)*, and wild cranesbill *(Geranium maculatum)*. Take twice daily in 5 ml doses.

   Yarrow tea: *Steep 1 to 2 tsp of the dried herb in 1 cup boiling water for 10 to 15 minutes. Drink up to 3 cups a day.*

YARROW

TIP *845*

PREVENTING OVARIAN CYSTS

To help prevent ovarian cysts, some alternative healthcare practitioners recommend a vegetarian diet rich in foods believed to nourish the liver, especially beets, carrots, dark-green leafy vegetables, and lemons. Others prescribe supplements of zinc and vitamins A, E, and C.

TIP *846*

ANTICYST HERBS

To help treat noncancerous ovarian cysts, try supplements of black currant oil, borage oil, or evening primrose oil *(Oenothera biennis);* all are believed to help regulate the body's hormone levels.

TIP *847*

ANTI-PID HERBS

To help fight pelvic inflammatory disease (PID) infection, herbalists recommend echinacea *(Echinacea* spp.*)* or calendula *(Calendula officinalis)*. Both of these herbs are believed to have antimicrobial properties. You may take these herbs in either tea or tincture form. (**Caution:** Because PID can lead to serious complications, such as infertility, never use these herbs as substitutes for conventional antibiotics. Consult your healthcare practitioner.)

ECHINACEA

TIP *848*

PID AND IUDS

Do not use an intrauterine device (IUD) for contraception.
Women wearing an IUD are three to five times more likely
to get PID than those not wearing one, especially if they have
more than one partner.

TIP *849*

TAKE PID PRECAUTIONS

Avoid putting anything in your vagina for two to three weeks
after an abortion, a miscarriage, or a dilation and curettage
(D&C) operation, and for six weeks after childbirth. This means
no intercourse, no douching, and no tampons. You should also
avoid bathing and swimming during this period; take showers
or sponge baths instead.

TIP *850*

HERBS FOR MORNING SICKNESS

To help ease the nausea during pregnancy that is commonly called
morning sickness, try teas made from anise *(Pim-*
pinella anisum), caraway *(Carum carvi)*, catnip
(Nepeta cataria), fennel *(Foeniculum vulgare)*, or
freshly grated ginger *(Zingiber officinale)*. An infusion
of dried peppermint *(Mentha piperita)* and chamomile
(Matricaria recutita) may also help ease your symptoms.

PEPPERMINT

TIP *851*

A CAUTION FOR
PREGNANT WOMEN

If you're a woman who is pregnant or planning to have a baby, get tested for chlamydia, even if you have no symptoms. Infected infants can develop conjunctivitis, a serious eye disease that could result in blindness.

TIP *852*

A STRONGER WOMB

To strengthen your uterus during pregnancy, try these gentle yoga exercises.

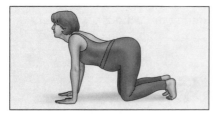

Get on your hands and knees, keeping your back flat. Inhale as you arch your back downward, keeping your head and buttocks raised. Hold this position for 10 seconds, then relax and breathe normally.

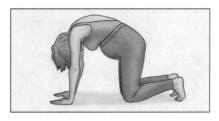

Next, exhale as you arch your back upward, rounding your shoulders and upper spine. Hold this position for 10 seconds, and then relax and breathe normally. Slowly repeat this up-and-down sequence 10 times.

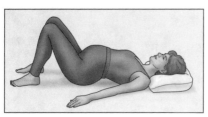

Lie on your back with your knees up. Tighten your buttocks and lower abdominal muscles, pressing the small of your back to the floor. Hold the position for 20 seconds, then relax and rest for one minute. Repeat five times.

TIP *853*

ANTI-PMS VITAMINS

Some PMS symptoms—including mood swings, fluid retention, bloatedness, breast tenderness, food cravings, and fatigue—have been linked to deficiencies of vitamin B_6 or the mineral magnesium. Nutritionists recommend supplements of these nutrients: 50 to 100 mg of vitamin B_6 daily, and 250 mg of magnesium daily, with a gradual increase if necessary. Supplements of calcium, zinc, copper, vitamins A and E, as well as various amino acids and enzymes are also sometimes prescribed.

TIP *854*

A DANDY REMEDY

In order to reduce the bloating and breast swelling caused by premenstrual fluid retention, try dandelion *(Taraxacum officinale)* tea.

Tea: *Simmer 2 to 3 tsp of the dried root in 1 cup of water for 15 minutes; drink three times a day.*

DANDELION

TIP *855*

A PRIMROSE PRIMER

Some research has shown that the essential fatty acids contained in evening primrose oil *(Oenothera biennis)* can relieve symptoms associated with premenstrual syndrome (PMS). Try one capsule (500 mg) daily throughout the month. If this amount does not bring relief, increase the dosage to 4 capsules a day. In Europe, women take 500 mg capsules of the oil two to three times a day for the relief of noncancerous breast pain and lumps. (Do not use evening primrose oil, however, if there is a chance you may be pregnant.)

TIP *856*

GET YOUR ZZZZZ'S

Lack of sleep can exacerbate irritability and other emotional symptoms associated with PMS. If you have trouble getting enough rest, stick to a regular sleep schedule. By going to bed and awakening at the same time each day, even on weekends, you may find it easier to get the sleep you need.

TIP *857*

DON'T DO DIURETICS

Although fluid retention—and the bloated feeling that accompanies it—is a common symptom of PMS, turning to diuretics for relief may not be not a good idea. Diuretics drain valuable minerals out of your body as well as fluids. A better way to do away with premenstrual bloatedness is to restrict your intake of salt and alcohol, which cause your body to retain water in the first place. Or try dandelion *(Tasaxacum officinale)*, a natural diuretic, or the homeopathic remedy *Natrum Sulphuricum* (6x), which may help return fluid to your bloodstream.

TIP *858*

AN ABSORBING FACT

Toxic shock syndrome, a potentially fatal condition caused by an overgrowth of a bacterium, has been directly linked to the use of tampons, especially superabsorbent ones. You can greatly reduce your risk of developing the syndrome by using the least absorbent tampon that will control your menstrual flow. Also, minimize your use of tampons; alternate them with sanitary napkins during the day, and use napkins at night.

TIP *859*

DON'T DOUCHE

Douching, particularly with commercial products, can alter the pH balance in your vagina, leaving you more susceptible to various vaginal infections. If you feel you must douche after intercourse or your menstrual period, use a diluted vinegar solution: Add 1 tbsp of white vinegar to the water container of your douche kit; then follow directions on the kit's label.

TIP *860*

A SALTY SITZ BATH

At the first signs of a mild vaginal infection—itching, irritation, or a change in the thickness or color of your vaginal discharge—take nightly saltwater sitz baths (½ cup table salt per bathtub of water). The salt water will help kill the offending bacteria. A sitz bath is simply a bath in which you immerse yourself only up to about the level of your navel.

TIP *861*

HOMEOPATHY FOR VAGINAL PROBLEMS

The following remedies taken three or four times a day for one or two days may be used for minor vaginal problems:

- *Kreosotum* (12c) for a smelly, yellow discharge with severe burning, swelling, and soreness.
- *Sepia* (12c) for itching and a white or yellow discharge.
- *Pulsatilla* (12c) for a thick, creamy yellow-green discharge.

See a professional homeopath if your condition does not clear up.

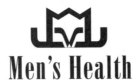

Men's Health

Practical

INFO ON

MEN'S HEALTH

ISSUES—FROM

IMPOTENCE AND

INFERTILITY TO

PROSTATE PROBLEMS

Men's Health

TIP *862*

BEAT THE HEAT
About 40 percent of infertility cases trace to problems with a man's sperm count or function. High temperature in the testicles can temporarily reduce sperm production; if you're trying to father a child, avoid saunas, hot tubs, and tight underwear.

TIP *863*

BIG TROUBLE FROM TINY VEINS
Varicoceles, or varicose veins in the scrotum, are sometimes the culprit behind male infertility. Up to 15 percent of adult men have varicoceles, which are almost always on the left side. Pain is rare, but discomfort can occur after hard exercise or prolonged standing. Most require no treatment, but if you have pain or suspect they may be impairing your fertility, see a urologist for help.

TIP *864*

BE ALERT TO TESTICULAR CANCER
Testicular cancer, the most common cancer in males 15 to 35 years old, mostly affects only one testicle. So, periodic checking that both are the same size and shape can help you catch any changes early. Other early warning signs include:
- a firm, initially painless lump.
- a feeling of testicular heaviness.
- urinary problems.
- abdominal mass or pain.
- persistent coughing, sometimes producing blood.
- shortness of breath.
- tenderness in the nipples, and breast enlargement.

TIP *865*

PRESCRIPTIONS FOR IMPOTENCE

Sometimes the cure for one ailment is the cause of another. A
number of drugs—including blood-pressure medicines, antidepressants, ulcer drugs, cholesterol-lowering agents, over-the-
counter decongestants, and antihistamines—can reduce blood
flow to the penis, resulting in impotence. But don't stop taking
medicine on your own; consult your doctor, who can usually
prescribe an alternative that doesn't cause this side effect.

TIP *866*

ANOTHER REASON NOT TO SMOKE

Because nicotine is a powerful vasoconstrictor, men who daily
smoke a pack of cigarettes or more drastically reduce the blood
circulation in their penile arteries. This, in turn, makes it difficult
if not impossible to achieve an erection. In many cases, blood
flow—along with sexual function—returns to normal in men who
kick the smoking habit.

TIP *867*

HERBAL SOLUTIONS FOR IMPOTENCE

Men with mild to moderate impotence may get a lift from yohim-
bine, a drug extracted from the bark of an African tree, or
from the prescription drug pentoxifylline, taken an
hour or two before intercourse. Some alternative practitioners recommend the Chinese herb golden cham-
ber (with or without cibot root). Other herbal therapies include ginkgo *(Ginkgo biloba)*, damiana *(Turnera*   GINKGO
diffusa), and Asian ginseng *(Panax ginseng)*.

TIP *868*

GET BACK IN CIRCULATION

Researchers have found that vasodilating drugs such as papaverine and prostaglandin can restore erectile function even in men who have been impotent for years. The drugs are typically administered by small-gauge injection or through a microsuppository inserted in the urethra. Regular use may improve long-term penile circulation and potency. Ask your physician or a urologist to explain which option may work for you.

TIP *869*

SQUEEZE PLAY

Try the "squeeze" technique to control premature ejaculation. When you feel that ejaculation is imminent, withdraw your penis and manually squeeze the glans, or tip, with the thumb and forefinger. This prevents climax by blocking blood flow to the glans. After 20 or 30 seconds, begin lovemaking again, repeating the squeeze several more times before proceeding to ejaculation. Over time, this technique can give you significantly greater natural control.

TIP *870*

DON'T IGNORE
A STRANGULATED HERNIA

In severe cases, an inguinal hernia may become strangulated, cutting off the blood supply to the protruding intestinal tissue. If you know you have a hernia and find yourself nauseated, vomiting, or unable to pass gas or have a bowel movement, seek a doctor's help immediately: A strangulated hernia is a medical emergency. Don't be misled by size, either. Small hernias are actually more likely to become strangulated than larger ones.

TIP 871

PREVENTING HERNIA

If you've had an inguinal hernia that has been surgically repaired, you are at greater risk of another. You can lower that risk by practicing these methods of reducing strain on your abdominal wall:

- If you are obese, lose weight.
- Include plenty of fiber in your diet to avoid constipation, and avoid straining during bowel movements.
- When picking up heavy objects, always lift from your knees, not your waist. Don't hold your breath, either; exhale as you lift.

TIP 872

HEED PROSTATE CANCER SIGNS

If you experience a frequent need to urinate, difficulty in starting or stopping the urine stream, pain when urinating or ejaculating, or blood in the urine or semen, see your doctor right away. These are signs of a swollen and possibly cancerous prostate, the walnut-sized gland that surrounds the urethra like a doughnut and helps produce semen. Other symptoms that may develop over time include back or bone pain, fatigue, loss of appetite, and nausea.

TIP 873

ATTENTION, MEN OVER 50

Some 200,000 American men are diagnosed with prostate cancer each year, and 38,000 of them die from the disease. At particular risk are African Americans, who are the most likely to get the disease. All men over the age of 50, but particularly African Americans, need to watch for signs of prostate trouble and have regular checkups. A good test for prostate cancer involves measuring the blood levels of a protein called prostate-specific antigen (PSA).

TIP*874*

ESCHEW THE FAT

Alhough the causes of prostate cancer are not well-understood, many experts now agree that one likely risk factor is high dietary fat, particularly when this fat comes from red meat or other animal sources. Researchers speculate that animal fats stimulate the production of testosterone and other male hormones, which in turn, fuel the growth and multiplication of cancerous cells in the prostate.

TIP*875*

YOGA

If you have an enlarged prostate, try the yoga position known as the Cobra.

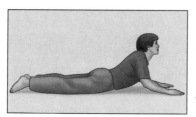

Cobra

Place both forearms on the floor, elbows directly under your shoulders. Inhale and push your chest up while pressing your pelvis against the ground. Hold for 15 seconds, breathing deeply, then slowly relax.

TIP*876*

PREVENTIVE MEASURES

To prevent a recurrence of chronic prostatitis, a bacterial infection of the prostate, and promote prostate health, try the following:

- Take warm sitz baths.
- Drink more water; dehydration stresses the prostate.
- Avoid prolonged bicycle riding, horseback riding, or other exercises that irritate the region below the prostate.
- Take supplements of zinc and vitamin C.

TIP *877*

ITCHING FOR RELIEF?

Jock itch, or *tinea cruris*, is a common fungal infection of a man's groin. In most cases, over-the-counter ointments containing miconazole or clotrimazole will clear up the problem. Chronic infections may require prescription drugs. To ensure curing the infection, continue applying antifungals for a month after the rash has gone.

TIP *878*

FOR KINDER CUTS

Men with moderate to severe acne should use a new razor blade every time they shave to lower the risk of infection. Instead of alcohol-based aftershaves, try soothing herbal alternatives such as the essential oil of lavender *(Lavandula officinalis)*, chamomile *(Matricaria recutita)*, or tea tree (*Melaleuca* spp.).

TIP *879*

TOO CLOSE FOR COMFORT?

If you have painful ingrown facial hairs, don't shave too closely. Use an electric shaver or a single-track razor instead of the double-blade variety, which cuts the hair off below skin level and encourages the whisker to double back into the skin.

TIP *880*

ICE AND HEAT TO THE RESCUE

If exercise or a hard day's work has left you stiff and sore, try icing the affected tissues. A bag of frozen vegetables works great as an ice pack; just be sure to put a damp towel around it first. The next day, you can use a warm compress along with proper stretching to ready yourself for a resumption of activity.

TIP *881*

HAIR TOMORROW?

The most common cause for hair loss in men is a condition called male-pattern baldness, which begins with a receding hairline then proceeds to the crown. "Cures" have been around since antiquity, but the first remedy that actually seems to help is a blood-pressure drug called minoxidil, recently approved by the FDA as a topical medication. Minoxidil works best on men who are just beginning to lose hair and does little for those who are already bald. Ask your doctor about the possible benefits and side effects of minoxidil.

TIP *882*

IF YOU CAN'T PERFORM, REHEARSE!

Failure to achieve or sustain an erection during sex leads to self-doubts and the need to "prove" oneself the next time. But the challenge sometimes only creates anxiety that makes performance all the more difficult. If you find yourself in this self-defeating spiral, try this: Forget about erections and focus on sensual touching instead. Partners who proceed with patience and learn how to give pleasure to each other without intercourse often find that potency returns naturally once the pressure to perform is off.

TIP *883*

WHEN A LOW BLOW
HAS YOU DOWN

Trauma to the testicles can cause severe pain, swelling, and discoloration sometimes accompanied by nausea and vomiting. A physician can usually determine via ultrasound whether a testicle has actually ruptured and requires surgical repair. If no rupture is found, the cause for discoloration may be internal bleeding. A sitz bath and bed rest with the scrotum elevated can help. You can also try the homeopathic remedy *Arnica* three times a day.

TIP *884*

HIDDEN DANGERS
OF IMPOTENCE

Doctors believe that most cases of chronic impotence, especially in men under 50, have a physical cause and in some cases may signal a serious disease, such as atherosclerosis or diabetes. See your physician, who has a variety of treatment options not only for your sexual problem but for many of the diseases that often underlie it.

TIP *885*

BETTER TO BE "B"

If you're an angry, hard-driving man, you may be driving yourself to a heart attack. In 1964, Drs. Meyer Friedman and Ray Rosenman linked certain personality traits to an increased risk for heart attacks. So-called Type A men are hurried, ambitious, and quick-tempered. Type B men, on the other hand, are laid back, easygoing, and unflappable. More recently, researchers have pegged two specific Type A characteristics—free-floating hostility and high levels of stress hormones in the blood—as particularly dangerous. The best advice: Slow down, mellow out, and if you must "drive" yourself anywhere, make it from A to B.

TIP *886*

SMELLS FOR SUCCESS

Practitioners of aromatherapy have found that the right combination of sensual scents can help a man relax and boost his ability to achieve erections. Use 4 tsp of massage oil and add 2 drops each of the essential oil of clary (*Salvia* spp.), sandalwood (*Cananga odorata*), and ylang-ylang (*Santalum album*). You can also add the oils to a warm bath.

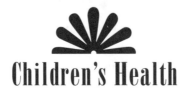

Children's Health

FROM INFANCY

TO THE

TEEN YEARS—TAKING

CARE OF YOUR

CHILDREN WITH THE

BEST CONVENTIONAL

TREATMENTS AND

NATURAL ALTERNATIVES

Children's Health

TIP 887

BABY STEPS

Children develop at different rates, but in general you can expect a two-week-old baby to maintain eye contact, a six-month-old to be able to sit up (with help), and an eight-month-old to begin crawling; around their first birthday, most children are taking a few steps and uttering simple words. If a child lags significantly in these motor and vocal skills, consult your doctor.

TIP 888

A COLIC CHECKLIST

If your baby begins to exhibit signs of colic, call your doctor to rule out other medical conditions. Also seek medical help if colic is accompanied by fever, diarrhea, or vomiting; if the baby is not gaining weight; or if colic persists after three months.

TIP 889

A CRY FOR HELP

Do not ignore a colicky baby; doctors now recommend that you take prompt action to relieve the crying bouts. Some things to try:

- Wrap the baby snugly in a blanket to provide a sense of security.
- Rock the baby, take him for a car ride, or put him in an infant seat near a clothes dryer, where he can feel the vibration.
- Place the baby, stomach down, on a warm hot-water bottle on your lap.

TIP *890*

THE GAS LINE

If colic seems related to meals, feed smaller amounts, more frequently; hold the baby upright and burp her often. If you are breast-feeding, eliminate milk, caffeine, broccoli, and cabbage from your own diet; these substances can be gas producing. Use a milk-free formula if you are bottle-feeding.

TIP *891*

CRIB SAFETY

Alhough doctors still do not know the cause of SIDS (Sudden Infant Death Syndrome), or crib death, it is thought that placing a baby on his back or side to sleep may reduce the risk. In addition, a baby should sleep on a firm mattress, without pillows, fluffy blankets, or stuffed animals.

TIP *892*

COUGH RELIEF

Mild cases of croup—raspy breathing, a barking cough—can generally be treated at home. To ease symptoms, try these remedies:
• Turn your bathroom into a steam room by turning on all the

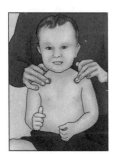

hot-water faucets. Take your child into the room until he breathes more easily. If the child is old enough, try to distract him by reading a story together.
   • For coughing spasms, try pressing on acupressure point Lung 1.

Place one finger of each hand about ½ inch below the large hollow under the collarbone, on the outer part of the chest near the shoulder. Press for one minute.

TIP *893*

MORE ACUPRESSURE RELIEF

To help calm a baby suffering from croup, try pressing the acupressure point known as Conception Vessel 17.

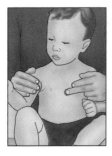

Conception Vessel 17
Place your finger in the center of the child's chest, midway between the nipples, and press lightly. Hold for one minute and release.

TIP *894*

WHEN CROUP IS A CRISIS

If your child has croup and is having extreme difficulty breathing, is turning pale or blue, or cannot speak or cry, call 911 or your emergency number. Do not tilt his head back to look inside his mouth; this could cause his throat to close completely, causing respiratory failure.

TIP *895*

FEBRILE SEIZURES

In infants and young children, a high fever—especially one that spikes, or rises very rapidly—can sometimes cause a seizure. If this occurs, remove the child's clothing and sponge her with lukewarm water; don't use cool or cold water or give the child a bath. Then call your doctor for further advice.

TIP 896

ROSEOLA:
IT'S NOT AS BAD AS IT LOOKS

Don't worry if your baby or toddler develops an itchless rash a few days after running a fever. Called roseola, the rash will clear up in a day or two, and requires no treatment.

TIP 897

DIARRHEA DANGER

Dehydration is a serious risk for infants and young children experiencing diarrhea. If a child has three or more runny bowel movements in a row, have him checked by a doctor as soon as possible.

TIP 898

DIAPER DOS

To avoid diaper rash, let your baby go bare as much as possible. When diapers are used, they should be changed as soon as they are damp or soiled. Cloth diapers should be washed in hot water with bleach, using extra rinse cycles to remove soap residue.

TIP 899

TEETHING PROBLEMS?
CHILL OUT

Stay away from over-the-counter teething medications, which can be toxic. Also dangerous is putting liquor on the gums. Instead, let your child chew on a chilled (not frozen) teething ring, or a chilled wet cloth. Or try rubbing calendula *(Calendula officinalis)* tincture on the gums to soothe and help heal them.

TIP *900*

AT FIRST BRUSH

When a child begins teething, start giving her gums and baby teeth a daily cleaning with gauze or a soft toothbrush. The first visit to a dentist should take place at the age of four.

TIP *901*

A POSITIVE APPROACH
TO THUMB-SUCKING

There's no reason to worry if your baby or toddler is a thumb-sucker; it's a harmless habit until a child starts getting his permanent teeth. At that point, you should use positive reinforcement to help your child break the habit.

- When you see your child sucking his thumb, draw his attention to what he is doing, but without being critical.
- Keep a calendar, and give the child a gold star for each day he goes without sucking his thumb.
- A week without thumb-sucking should be rewarded with a special treat.

TIP *902*

KEEP CALM OVER WET BEDS

Parents should never punish their children for bed-wetting, which is simply a sign of an immature bladder and is likely to resolve itself after a child reaches the age of six.

TIP *903*

EXERCISE FOR
BLADDER CONTROL

Children who wet the bed can increase their bladder capacity, making it easier for them to stay dry through the night, through a stretching exercise. Once a day, have your child hold his urine as long as possible after his body is telling him that it's time to go.

TIP *904*

ADENOIDS AND ALLERGIES

Symptoms of enlarged adenoids—open-mouthed breathing, recurrent ear infections—should be checked by a doctor. These can be indications that a child is suffering from allergies and may need a series of shots. In severe cases, where the child has intervals of not breathing during the night, surgery may be necessary.

TIP *905*

DOES IT ADD UP TO ADD?

Though some skeptics doubt its very existence, Attention Deficit Disorder has become the standard diagnosis for children who exhibit a cluster of behavioral problems, including inability to pay attention, disorganization, distractibility, impulsiveness, and hyperactivity. Children suspected of having ADD should be evaluated by someone who specializes in evaluating and treating the disorder. The standard treatment is the brand-name drug Ritalin, a stimulant that has the paradoxical effect of making ADD children calmer and better able to concentrate. But homeopathic practitioners also claim success using so-called constitutional remedies—ones that take into account the child's entire physical, mental, and emotional makeup.

TIP *906*

MEASLES

One of the most severe childhood diseases, measles—character-ized by a high fever and small red bumps that spread from the face to the torso and limbs—can be prevented by timely vaccina-tion. If your child does contract the disease, consult your doctor; you need to be on guard against potentially serious complica-tions. Children with measles should be kept in bed, both to help their bodies heal and to prevent them from spreading the infec-tion. If the eyes are affected, the lights in the child's room should be kept low. Also, consider consulting a homeopathic physician for remedies that may help speed your child's recovery.

TIP *907*

GERMAN MEASLES

With symptoms that are much milder than the measles—a low-grade fever, a less extensive rash, or no rash at all—German measles is not unlike a bad cold for most children, and can be treated accordingly: with rest, acetaminophen, and cool sponge baths. Children with the disease are contagious for about a week after the rash disappears, so during that time they should be kept away from other children and, particularly, pregnant women.

TIP *908*

AN AILMENT THAT'S
HARD TO SWALLOW

Though the mumps is a relatively mild infection, you should con-tact your doctor if your child comes down with it. Standard treat-ment includes rest, heat, or ice on the swelling, and a diet of light, soft foods. Avoid citrus fruits and juices, which can further irritate the affected salivary glands. For an easy-to-swallow bever-age, gently boil eight whole cloves in one quart apple juice, strain, and serve at room temperature.

TIP *909*

BLISTER BUSTERS

If you think your child has chickenpox (characterized by itchy red bumps that develop into blisters), call your doctor to confirm the diagnosis. The doctor may want to prescribe an antihistamine to relieve the painful itching. Antibiotics are necessary only if the lesions are oozing or inflamed; this indicates that a secondary infection has set in. Homeopathic remedies such as *Rhus toxicodendron* may speed healing; consult a homeopathic physician for the best remedy for your child.

TIP *910*

SOLVING A TOUCHY PROBLEM

It's not easy, but you should keep a child with chickenpox from scratching, since it can lead to infection and scarring. Trim fingernails and file them smooth, or disarm your child by putting him or her in mittens.

TIP *911*

ITCH RELIEF

Chickenpox sufferers can be soothed by lukewarm baths; add a handful of oatmeal or baking soda to the bathwater. Calamine or witch hazel, applied to the blisters, can also provide relief from itching. Do not use cortisone creams. Instead, place a combination of calendula *(Calendula officinalis)* and goldenseal *(Hydrastis canadensis)* ointments directly on the pox to reduce itching and speed healing without side effects.

GOLDENSEAL

TIP *912*

ASPIRIN ISN'T FOR CHILDREN

Never give aspirin to a child or an adolescent suffering from the flu or other viral infection such as chicken pox: Its use is associated with a potentially fatal complication called Reye's syndrome. Symptoms of the syndrome (which can afflict children even if they have not taken aspirin) include confusion, persistent vomiting, and extreme fatigue. If these occur, get immediate medical help.

TIP *913*

THE RED FLAG OF SCARLET FEVER

If your child develops scarlet fever—rough red patches on the neck and chest, accompanied by a high fever—get immediate medical help. Scarlet fever cannot be left to run its course like some other childhood illnesses. It must be treated with antibiotics to avoid serious complications such as arthritis and kidney problems.

TIP *914*

FIGHTING FATIGUE WITH HERBS

Teas made from ginseng, either Aisian *(Panax ginseng)* or the American *(Panax quinquefolius)* form, can help relieve the fatigue that can persist for months after an acute attack of mononucleosis. St.-John's-wort *(Hypericum perforatum)* may alleviate the depression that can accompany the disease.

GINSENG

TIP *915*

BOYHOOD GROWTH

If a boy has not had a significant growth spurt by the age of 15, or he is 16 and his voice has not begun to change, schedule a visit with his doctor to discuss delayed puberty.

TIP 916

A MONTHLY BULLETIN

Girls generally begin menstruating between the ages of 11 and 14; if they have not begun by the age of 17, a visit to a gynecologist is in order. However, it often takes a few years for an adolescent to establish a regular cycle. Girls should have a pelvic exam by their 18th birthday, sooner if they are having severe menstrual problems or are sexually active.

TIP 917

REAL GROWING PAINS

An adolescent experiencing swelling and discomfort below the kneecap, unassociated with an injury, may literally be suffering from growing pains, also known as Osgood-Schlatter disease. In severe cases, the knee may be taped or otherwise immobilized. Milder cases can be treated with ice packs and ibuprofen, and by avoiding exercise that strains the knee.

TIP 918

DETECTING DEPRESSION

Puberty, with its raging hormones, typically transforms cheerful children into moody teenagers. But parents need to be aware that some adolescent angst is, in fact, clinical depression. Get psychiatric help if a teenager (or younger child) is suffering from persistent insomnia, fatigue, headache or stomach ache, has difficulty concentrating, is performing below par in school, has lost interest in friends and activities he or she previously enjoyed, or is abusing drugs or alcohol, or says he or she would be better off dead. Don't ignore these warning signs.

TIP *919*

STARVING FOR ATTENTION

A life-threatening eating disorder that generally occurs during adolescence, anorexia nervosa requires prompt medical intervention. The disorder commonly affects girls, although boys are not immune, and is characterized by obsession with body image, eating rituals, and dieting carried to dangerous extremes. Treatment includes antidepressant and antianxiety medications, as well as behavioral and family therapy.

TIP *920*

ANOREXIA AND EXERCISE

Exercise such as yoga, t'ai chi, dance, and swimming can help reduce anxiety and improve body image in anorexics. But any physical activities program should be supervised, since anorexics sometimes exercise compulsively in order to accelerate their weight loss.

TIP *921*

THE SUBTLE
SIGNS OF BULIMIA

A disorder that is related to anorexia nervosa, and sometimes exists in tandem with it, bulimia—the practice of bingeing on foods, then inducing vomiting—also requires prompt medical assistance. Since bulimics may maintain a normal weight, parents should be alert to the signs, which include consumption of large quantities of food, immediately followed by a visit to the bathroom; abuse of laxatives; and tooth discoloration and other dental problems (caused by the damaging effects of the acids in vomit).

TIP *922*

NUTRITIONAL THERAPY

Bulimics on the road to recovery should eat balanced, nutrient-dense meals, supplemented by a multivitamin along with additional vitamin C and B complex. They should avoid sugar, alcohol, caffeine, salt, and cigarettes.

TIP *923*

SAVING FACE

Mild adolescent acne can usually be managed with over-the-counter remedies like benzoyl peroxide creams. But to avoid physical and psychological scarring, a teen should consult a dermatologist if breakouts are severe. Antibiotics, both oral and topical, can be very effective in clearing up acne. An herbal acne preparation made from the calendula *(Calendula officinalis)* flower is also helpful. CALENDULA

TIP *924*

CHOCOLATE IS
NOT THE PROBLEM

Avoiding chocolate and greasy French fries—traditionally pegged as acne instigators—probably won't beneficially affect your teenager's acne. Iodine, however, may make acne worse; sources of iodine include beef liver, broccoli, table salt, and onions, as well as many multivitamin supplements. Helpful nutritional supplements include vitamins E, A, and B_6, chromium, and especially, zinc; consult a doctor or nutritionist for safe dosages.

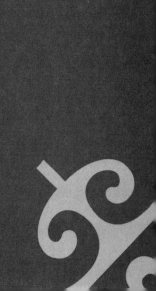

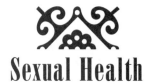

Sexual Health

STRAIGHTFORWARD

ADVICE FOR

MEN AND WOMEN

ON HOW TO STAY

SEXUALLY HEALTHY

AND HAPPY

Sexual Health

TIP 925

AN OYSTER A DAY . . .

Zinc seems to play a role in hormonal activity in both men and women. To keep reproductive systems healthy—and to help combat sexually transmitted diseases—take a 22 to 25 mg capsule of zinc daily. Natural sources of zinc are oysters, wheat bread, oatmeal, and pumpkin and sunflower seeds.

TIP 926

SYMPTOMS NOT TO IGNORE

Seek immediate medical help for any unusual vaginal or penile discharge, pain or bleeding during sex, or any genital rash, blisters or warts, even if these do not cause discomfort. These can be symptoms of a sexually transmitted disease, and must be treated to protect your own health and that of your partner.

TIP 927

KEEP CHLAMYDIA IN CHECK

Sexually active women, especially those with more than one partner, should be checked regularly for chlamydia, an extremely common bacterial disease spread through intercourse. Testing is crucial because chlamydia is generally asymptomatic in women. Many women discover that they have been infected only when they develop pelvic inflammatory disease, a serious complication that can result in sterility. Caught early, chlamydia responds very well to antibiotics and sulfa drugs.

TIP *928*

HERPES: FOOD DOS AND DON'TS

The herpes virus needs the amino acid arginine to thrive, so
people with herpes should avoid arginine-rich foods
such as peanuts, cashews, and chocolate. Conversely,
the amino acid lysine inhibits the growth of the virus,
so it's a good idea to consume beef, lamb, fish, milk, and
cheese, which have an abundance of lysine. Lysine can also be
taken in capsule form; 500 mg is the recommended daily dose.

TIP *929*

WORRYING ONLY MAKES THINGS WORSE

Since stress can make the outbreaks of herpes or genital warts
more frequent and more severe, try to stay calm. Relaxation
techniques such as meditation, self-hypnosis or massage can
help. You can buy cassettes that guide you into meditation, or
consult a hypnotherapist.

TIP *930*

GET RELIEF WITH TEA TREE OIL

A potent germicide, tea tree oil (*Melaleuca* spp.), available at
health food stores, can help heal genital warts or the blisters
of genital herpes. The oil can also be used in a douche for
minor vaginal problems. **Warning:** Tea tree oil can be irritating
to people with sensitive skin, who may need to dilute it with a
bland vegetable oil.

TIP *931*

THE VALUE OF GOLDENSEAL

An herb with antiseptic and anti-inflammatory properties, goldenseal *(Hydrastis canadensis)* has a variety of sexual-health benefits. Women who are prone to bladder infections can prevent recurrences by washing their genitals with a goldenseal solution before and after intercourse; goldenseal douches can help treat cervicitis; goldenseal tea can ameliorate the symptoms of moniliasis or gonorrhea.

GOLDENSEAL

Cleansing solution: Simmer 2 tsp goldenseal in a cup of water for 15 minutes; cool to room temperature. A douching solution should contain only half as much goldenseal.

Tea: Mix 2 to 3 tsp into a cup of boiling water; drink 3 cups a day.

TIP *932*

TIMING IT RIGHT

By observing the changes in her body during her monthly cycle, a woman can often tell when she's most likely to conceive. In the middle of the month, during ovulation, the vaginal mucus is thinner and clearer than it is during her infertile periods. If these changes do not occur, or if a drugstore ovulation kit comes up negative three months in a row, a woman trying to get pregnant should see her doctor.

TIP *933*

TREATING GENITAL WARTS

Over-the-counter wart medications are too strong to be used on
the genitals. See your doctor, who can "paint" the warts with a
chemical called podophyllin. The treatment is generally effective
within a few weeks.

TIP *934*

THE POWER OF GARLIC

With its antibacterial, antifungal, and antiviral properties, garlic
(Allium sativum) can be useful in treating a number of
reproductive-tract problems. Apply garlic oil to genital warts
with a cotton swab twice a day to help dry them up. To
help vaginal infections heal, douche with a mixture of
4 drops garlic oil and ¼ cup water; hold it for two or
three minutes, then expel. You can also consume garlic
in food or as tablets to help the body ward off all sorts of
other diseases and disorders.

GARLIC

TIP *935*

HELP FOR TRICHOMONIASIS

According to aromatherapists, women with trichomoniasis—a
parasitic infection that is transmitted sexually—can bathe or
douche with oil of bergamot *(Citrus bergamia)* to help dry up
the discharges.

TIP 936

PUTTING PRESSURE ON
GONORRHEA GERMS

Chinese medical practitioners advocate that people with gonorrhea stimulate their liver and kidneys with acupressure, to help
cleanse their systems and build up energy. (Note: This is not a
substitute for antibiotics.)

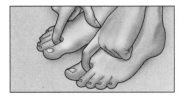

Liver 2
*On the top of each foot, use your index fin-
ger to press into the webbing between the big
toe and the second toe.*

TIP 937

A TIME TO FAST

Some experts believe that water or juice fasts may release a hormone that enhances the immune system, thereby helping the
body rid itself of infections, including sexually transmitted ones
like gonorrhea. But never begin a fast without first checking
with your healthcare practitioner.

TIP 938

TAKE A VACATION FROM SEX

Women suffering from vaginal or bladder infections, whether
or not they are sexually transmitted, should refrain from sexual
intercourse until the symptoms disappear. They should also
avoid intercourse—as well as douching, tampons, and tub baths
—for three weeks after an abortion, miscarriage, or D&C, and
for six weeks after childbrith.

TIP *939*

CONDOM BASICS

For protection against sexually transmitted diseases, use latex condoms, not the more porous ones made from animal skin. A water-based lubricant is safe, but avoid oil-based lubricants, such as petroleum jelly. The condom should be put on before the penis comes into contact with the vagina, mouth, or anus. To put on a condom: Unroll it over an erect penis, leaving space at the tip for semen to collect. After sex, hold the condom by the rim and pull it off slowly. Use a fresh condom for each act of intercourse.

TIP *940*

ALLERGIC REACTIONS

Condoms are crucial in preventing the spread of disease. But they can cause some health problems. Both men and women can have allergic reactions to latex; see your doctor if this occurs. Spermicides can also cause irritation. Putting a spermicide inside the tip of a condom, rather than on the outside, can help if the woman is the one who reacts badly to the chemicals.

TIP *941*

DIAPHRAGM DIAGNOSTICS

A diaphragm that doesn't fit properly can make a woman more susceptible to bladder infections. Have your doctor check yours regularly, particularly if you've gained or lost weight. If you're prone to recurrent infections, consider using another form of birth control.

TIP *942*

PROTECTIVE DEVICES

A woman's choice of contraception can make her more or less vulnerable to cervical problems and pelvic inflammatory disease (PID). These conditions arise when the cervix and uterus are exposed to disease organisms in semen; women should use contraceptive methods—condoms, diaphragms, or cervical caps— that shield them from potential pathogens. Since intrauterine devices (IUDs) more than triple the chance of contracting PID (either sudden and acute, or chronic and low level), they are best avoided.

TIP *943*

SMOKEFREE FOR FERTILITY

Kick the smoking habit if you want to make a baby. Studies have shown that men who smoke have lower sperm counts and less sperm motility. Smoking can also alter a woman's hormonal balance, making her less fertile.

TIP *944*

CONCEPTION MADE SIMPLE

The missionary position is best for couples trying to get pregnant. After sex, the woman should continue lying on her back for at least 20 minutes; this makes it easier for the sperm to make their way into the uterus.

TIP 945

WATCH YOUR WEIGHT
BEFORE YOU GET PREGNANT

A woman is most likely to get pregnant if she keeps her weight close to what's recommended for her height and body frame. Too much or too little body fat can cause a hormonal imbalance that impairs fertility.

TIP 946

DON'T OVERDO IT

Once is all it takes to get pregnant. But once a day can be too much of a good thing. It takes time for sperm to build up again after ejaculation, so every other day is the best schedule for couples hoping to get pregnant.

TIP 947

SAFE SEX
DURING PREGNANCY

Contrary to popular belief, couples can safely enjoy intercourse until close to the baby's due date. However, a woman should check with her doctor if she has a history of miscarriage or preterm birth, if the placenta is in an abnormal position, if there is any bleeding or sign of infection, or if she is carrying multiple fetuses.

TIP *948*

A NATURAL LUBRICANT
FOR CONCEPTION

For a natural way to combat vaginal dryness during intercourse, look no further than your refrigerator. Egg white—at room temperature—makes an excellent vaginal lubricant. And for couples hoping to get pregnant, there is evidence that egg whites, unlike commercial lubricants, will not kill or impede sperm.

TIP *949*

FOR WOMEN OF A CERTAIN AGE

Sexual desire does not necessarily diminish after menopause; many women find that it increases. Vaginal dryness associated with lower levels of estrogen, however, can make intercourse difficult. A diet rich in foods that are high in plant estrogens, such as soybeans, lima beans, celery, parsley, fennel, and nuts, might help. So might tea made from the herb black cohosh *(Cimicifuga racemosa).* And applying either vitamin E oil or the Bach flower Rescue Remedy twice a day can also

BLACK COHOSH   greatly decrease vaginal dryness.

TIP *950*

A CHANGE OF
POSITION CAN HELP

Although a tipped uterus is generally nothing to worry about, it can cause sexual difficulties: The penis bumps into the uterus, making intercourse painful for the woman. This problem can often be averted by having the woman crouch on her hands and knees, while the man enters her from behind.

TIP 951

IMPOTENCE:
IT ISN'T ALL IN THE MIND

Doctors now realize that many cases of impotence (the chronic form, not the occasional episodes that all men experience) have a physiological, rather than a psychological, cause. How to tell which is which? If you have early-morning erections, or are able to masturbate, problems with a partner are almost certainly psychological in origin; counseling or sex therapy can help. If not, particularly if you are over 50, the difficulty you are having could be the result of narrowing of the penile artery or other physical disorder or disease. See a urologist, who may prescribe medication or implants. And be aware that various medications, including drugs to treat high blood pressure and depression, can dampen desire. A new prescription may be all that's needed.

TIP 952

HELP FOR
PREMATURE EJACULATORS

Although a prostate infection or neurological disorder can some-times cause premature ejaculation, the problem is generally psychological in nature. After physical causes have been ruled out, the standard treatment is a highly effective form of biofeedback known as the squeeze technique. When a man is about to climax, he (or his partner) gently squeezes the head of the penis between the thumb and forefinger for 20 seconds. Repeat several times in the course of making love.

TIP 953

CLEANLINESS IS NEXT TO . . .

To help prevent "honeymoon cystitis"—the bladder infection that afflicts many sexually active women, particularly those engaging in frequent or vigorous intercourse—women should wash their sexual organs and empty their bladders both before and after intercourse, to keep bacteria from being pushed into the urethra. Men should follow their example.

TIP 954

UNSCENTED IS BEST

Many cases of irritation of the vulva and vagina are the result of exposure to the perfumes and dyes in a variety of ordinary products. Women prone to these problems should avoid feminine hygiene sprays, perfumed douches, scented tampons, and colored toilet paper. Certain soaps, bath oil, spermicides, and lubricants can also be irritating to some women.

TIP 955

THE ONLY SAFE
USE FOR SPANISH FLY

Highly irritating to the bladder, *Cantharis* (Spanish fly) was once believed—wrongly—to have aphrodisiac qualities. In homeopathic medicine, however, extremely dilute quantities are used to treat bladder infections.

TIP 956

THE RELAXING EFFECTS OF SEX

One of the best remedies for PMS, menstrual cramps, or the perturbations of pregnancy is making love. Aside from giving women a chance to focus on pleasure rather than pain, sex—especially orgasmic sex—relieves congestion in the pelvis, and relaxes tense muscles throughout the body.

TIP 957

DO YOUR KEGELS

Women can learn to become more orgasmic by exercising their vaginal muscles with so-called Kegel exercises. After urination, contract your pelvic floor muscles and hold for 10 seconds. Repeat several times. Kegel exercises also help with incontinence and a prolapsed uterus.

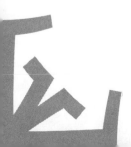

Mental Health

FROM PROBLEMS

YOU CAN TREAT

YOURSELF—TO WHEN

AND HOW

TO GET HELP FOR

YOURSELF OR

A LOVED ONE

———————

Mental Health

TIP 958

STRENGTH IN NUMBERS

When feeling overwhelmed by a problem, resist the urge to withdraw and instead enlist the aid of a friend, counselor, or member of the clergy. With a little help, seemingly insurmountable problems become much easier to cope with and overcome.

TIP 959

PRESS THE UN-PANIC BUTTON

To reduce the severity of an anxiety attack, press your index finger or thumb at the point above your upper lip that's directly below your nose. Keep the pressure steady on this so-called antispasmodic point for one minute.

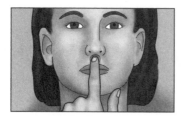

Governing Vessel 26
With your index finger or thumb, press firmly on this point, which is two-thirds of the way up from the upper lip to the nose.

TIP 960

BREATHING OUT ANXIETY

If anxiety leads you to hyperventilate, try breathing through your nose. If you still feel faint or dizzy, breathe through cupped hands or into a paper bag.

TIP *961*

RESISTANCE:
THE WRONG APPROACH

To triumph over panic, stop fighting it and accept it. The more you resist and "awful-ize" the symptoms, the more they will persist. Instead of saying, "I want to avoid these feelings at all costs," tell yourself, "I want to face the symptoms so that I can learn to gain better coping skills."

TIP *962*

PRACTICE PATIENCE

When anxiety strikes, float with your feelings and let time pass. Don't be impatient; the less you try to rush away the unpleasant feelings, the more quickly they will recede.

TIP *963*

ANXIETY REMEDIES

Proponents of Bach flower essences recommend several remedies to help diminish the symptoms of anxiety. The best include Rescue Remedy, Aspen, and Mimulus. The homeopathic remedy *Aconite* is also said to be an excellent treatment for anxiety and panic attacks. Consult a practitioner for dosages.

TIP *964*

ORGANIC ROOTS

If you suffer anxiety symptoms that you can't manage, ask your doctor to rule out possible organic diseases. Hyperthyroidism (an overactive thyroid), hyper- or hypocalcemia (too much or too little calcium), tachycardia (rapid heart rate), hypoglycemia (low blood sugar), and other conditions can sometimes cause the same symptoms as an anxiety disorder.

TIP *965*

DEFINITIVE DIAGNOSIS

When you decide you need help, see a physician specializing in emotional disorders for a diagnosis of your problem. A host of treatment options exists, and an accurate diagnosis is the first step in creating a personalized treatment plan of counseling, medication, or both.

TIP *966*

TAILOR-MADE THERAPY

Do some research to discover the form—or forms—of therapy that will best help you cope with your anxiety. Different people respond better to different therapies. Behavior modification, cognitive therapy, traditional "talk" psychotherapy, and other disciplines provide a wide array of choices.

TIP *967*

MEDICAL ADJUNCT

If your anxiety is impairing your ability to function, ask your doctor about antianxiety medicines. In some cases, short-term treatment with the class of drugs known as benzodiazepines can help patients make more rapid progress in therapy. Also ask about buspirone, a promising new antianxiety drug that lacks many of the benzodiazepines' side effects and potential for dependency.

TIP *968*

CALMING BRAIN WAVES

If anxiety causes both physical and mental symptoms, try learning EEG (electroencephalogram) biofeedback. The noninvasive monitoring device allows you to see the waves your brain produces. Many patients can learn in about a dozen sessions how to consciously calm anxious brain waves, at which point they no longer need the EEG monitor.

TIP *969*

HYPNOSIS FOR PHOBIAS

Ask a qualified hypnotherapist to teach you self-hypnosis to conquer phobias like stage fright or fear of exams. Despite its sinister reputation in movies, hypnosis is not a magical form of mind control but rather a form of deeply relaxed concentration. Patients who learn self-hypnosis can also calm more generalized anxiety.

TIP 970

NO SHAME

Do not give in to shame or the belief that emotional problems are a sign of weakness. Share your situation with close friends and relatives. They will almost certainly admire your openness—and may even be moved to share their own problems with you.

TIP 971

PRACTICE IMPERFECTIONISM

When learning new coping skills for emotional disorders, give yourself permission to fail. Whether you're trying biofeedback or a new medication, don't say to yourself, "This had better be 100 percent effective." Instead say: "It's OK if it doesn't work—I'll keep trying till I find something that does help me."

TIP 972

SUSPECT THE SUGAR

If you suffer panic attacks, try a preliminary self-test for hypoglycemia (low blood sugar), which can cause identical symptoms. When an attack strikes, drink fruit juice or eat a candy bar. If the symptoms markedly diminish within 30 minutes, see your doctor for more comprehensive blood sugar testing.

TIP 973

MEDICINAL RELIEF

Try to view medications in a realistic light. A variety of current drugs do offer substantial relief to many patients suffering from emotional disorders, and promising new medicines are coming on line every year. Still, there are no "magic pills." Even the best medicines can only help you believe in your personal control over your body and life.

TIP 974

CHECK THOSE RITUALS

If you suffer from the involuntary and persistent thoughts or rituals that are the hallmark of obsessive-compulsive disorder (OCD), consult a psychiatrist who can combine drug treatment with behavior therapy. Antidepressant drugs such as the tricyclic antidepressant clomipramine and SSRIs (for "selective serotonin reuptake inhibitors") like fluoxetine, paroxetine, and sertraline can significantly reduce OCD symptoms, especially when supplemented with behavior therapy.

TIP 975

NO COMMENT

If you are a friend or relative of someone suffering from the eating disorder anorexia nervosa, refrain from commenting on weight, eating, grooming, or grades. Show instead that you value the person's internal qualities.

TIP *976*

SUPPLEMENTAL ZINC

For someone with anorexia, ask the doctor about supplements of zinc sulfate. Zinc deficiency is particularly common in anorexics who are also vegetarians, and it can retard both growth and sexual development.

TIP *977*

MEDICINE FOR BULIMIA

See your doctor about medical treatment for the binge-and-purge eating disorder, bulimia. A class of antidepressant drugs known as SSRIs is now considered a mainstay of treatment along with psychological counseling.

TIP *978*

ALCOHOLIC ANXIETY

If you are dependent on alcohol and also suffer anxiety disorders, treat the alcoholism first by joining a group like Alcoholics Anonymous (AA). Up to one-quarter of men and women with long-term anxiety disorders become alcoholics as a way to "self-medicate" their symptoms. Once you get your chemical dependency under control, you will find it much easier to tackle the underlying anxiety.

ㅠㅍ*979*

ACUPUNCTURE
FOR ALCOHOLISM

To reduce withdrawal symptoms, prevent seizures, and lessen the risk of alcoholic relapse, seek the help of a licensed acupuncturist as an adjunct to your recovery program.

ㅠㅍ*980*

NONSPIRITUAL RECOVERY

For recovering alcoholics who object to the spiritual emphasis of 12-step support programs like Alcoholics Anonymous (AA), consider joining alternative groups such as Rational Recovery or Women for Sobriety.

ㅠㅍ*981*

SOBRIETY HERBS

To reduce alcoholic withdrawal symptoms, infuse 2 tsp of skullcap *(Scutellaria lateriflora)*, lavender *(Lavandula officinalis)*, or motherwort *(Leonurus cardiaca)* in water, and take three times a day. Or try the homeopathic mineral combination *biochemic phosphates;* taken four times a day, it may help to diminish withdrawal symptoms and promote relaxation.

SKULLCAP

TIP *982*

PUTTING THE TEA
INTO TREATMENT

Try an herbal tea to relax you on the road to recovery. Some alcoholism treatment centers recommend a sleep-mix tea made from equal parts chamomile *(Matricaria recutita)*, hops *(Humulus lupulus)*, skullcap *(Scutelleria lateriflora)*, peppermint *(Mentha piperita)*, yarrow *(Achillea millefolium)*, and either catnip *(Nepeta cataria)* or valerian *(Valeriana officinalis)*.

HOPS

TIP *983*

A NEW LIFE

To keep sober, avoid the drinking lifestyle. Find new friends, join a recovery group, and use exercise to get high naturally.

TIP *984*

EAT RIGHT TO STOP DRINKING

Consult a nutritionist for help in restoring vital nutrients, such as thiamine (vitamin B_1), that are often missing from the diets of alcoholics. A recent study found that proper nutritional therapy doubles the rate of recovery.

TIP *985*

TELLING NORMAL SADNESS FROM CLINICAL DEPRESSION

If you feel blue for more than two weeks, see your doctor to help distinguish between a depressive reaction that usually doesn't need treatment and a depressive illness that does. Minor, temporary depression affects almost everyone at some point, but if it is severe, long-lasting, or accompanied by symptoms like insomnia, weight loss or gain, anxiety, or loss of interest in sex, odds are you have a medical condition that can and should be treated.

TIP *986*

WHEN THE BLAHS PERSIST

Seek treatment for dysthymia. This chronic low-grade form of depression is not characterized by intense sadness or hopelessness, but rather by a persistent "blah" feeling that can last two years or longer. The good news: Dysthymia is highly treatable; see your healthcare practitioner to restore life to your life.

TIP *987*

SOLACE FROM ST. JOHN

Consult your doctor or an herbalist about drinking tea made from St.-John's-wort *(Hypericum perforatum)* to relieve depression. Studies show this herb, used properly, can be as effective as leading antidepressants.

Tea: *Add 1 to 2 tsp of the dried herb to 1 cup of boiling water; steep for 15 minutes. Drink up to 3 cups a day.*

St.-John's-Wort

TIP 988

LIGHTEN UP

Relieve depression by exposing yourself to natural sunlight during the day. Too little full-spectrum light during the daytime—or too much at night—can throw off your body's internal clock and leave you feeling tired and blue.

TIP 989

WINTER OF DISCONTENT

Move south—or at least take a southern vacation—if you suffer depression each winter. This condition, known as seasonal affective disorder (SAD), appears to be triggered in susceptible people by the low light of winter. Heading south to sunnier climes can make a real difference: SAD is up to eight times less likely to strike in Mexico than in Canada.

TIP 990

HEALING VOLTAGE

Although still controversial, electroconvulsive therapy (ECT) is not what it once was. In the last 20 years, advances in ECT have made this painless treatment for severe depression as safe as medications in some cases—and often more effective.

TIP 991

TAG TEAM CURE

Supplement drug therapy with short-term psychotherapy. Effective as medication can be at correcting the neurochemical imbalances that underlie depression, supportive talk therapy can bolster this effect by teaching you how to overcome negative attitudes, return to normal activities, and gain new coping skills.

TIP *992*

MODERATING MOOD SWINGS

If you suffer the intense agony-to-ecstasy mood swings character-
istic of manic depression, ask your doctor about treatment with
lithium carbonate, which can be remarkably effective in reducing
mania. It can also help prevent the recurrence of depression, although doctors often prescribe it in conjunction with other antidepressants.

TIP *993*

ACUPRESSURE RELIEF

Try acupressure at the Liver 8 point as an adjunct to—not a
replacement for—conventional treatments for depression.

Liver 8
*Bend the right knee and place your right
thumb just above the knee crease on the inside of the leg. The point lies just below the
knee joint (swing your leg a few times to help
locate it). Press, then repeat on the other leg.*

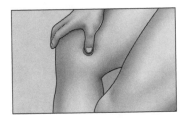

TIP 994

AEROBIC CURE

Exercise vigorously for 30 minutes three or more times a week. Studies show that physical exercise, the more energetic the better, can often moderate depression as effectively as psychotherapy. For some depressed patients, the mood-elevating effects of exercise can border on the miraculous.

TIP 995

INVIGORATING VITAMINS

If you're depressed, adopt a healthful diet and bolster it with supplements of vitamin B complex, folic acid (400 mcg daily), and S-adenosylmethionie (two 800 mg doses daily). Taking 50 mcg daily of selenium can also elevate your mood if your body is deficient in selenium.

TIP 996

AVOID THE CRASH

To avoid exacerbating your depression, stay away from alcohol, junk food, sugar, aspartame, and caffeine. Such substances may give you a short-lived spurt of energy or high feeling, but in the long run, they'll bring you down.

TIP 997

PRACTICE PROPHYLAXIS

Take steps to prevent recurrence of depression. Up to 75 percent of people who suffer a depressive illness will endure another bout within 10 years. But there's good evidence that you can beat the odds with a healthy lifestyle. Remind yourself always to eat well, exercise regularly, take vacations, don't overwork, and save time to do something fun.

TIP *998*

GIVE IT TIME

If your physician recommends antidepressant medication as part of your treatment plan, give it a fair trial. Many antidepressants, for example, can require a full month or longer to reach optimal effectiveness.

TIP *999*

TOO LITTLE WON'T HELP

Make sure to take the full dose of any medication your doctor recommends for any emotional problems. Taking an inadequate amount "to prove you don't really need it" is one of the most common reasons for drug-treatment failure.

TIP *1000*

WAIT OUT SIDE EFFECTS

Expect some side effects from psychoactive medications. These can range from dry mouth and blurred vision to difficulty in urinating and dizziness upon standing suddenly. These side effects should moderate over time; if they don't, let your doctor know.

TIP *1001*

FIND A CHEERLEADER

As you work to overcome an anxiety disorder, depression, or other mental health problem, enlist the aid of a reassuring supporter—someone who will remind you of the variety of effective coping methods, hail your success, and infect you with optimism about the future.

Picture & Art Credits

Credits from left to right are separated by semicolons; credits from top to bottom are separated by dashes.

Front Cover: ©Jackson Vereen/FoodPix--©1996 Paul Venning/Leo de Wys, Inc.; ©1996 Runk/Schoenberger/Grant Heilman Photography, Inc.

Back Cover: ©1996 Runk/Schoenberger/Grant Heilman Photography, Inc.-- ©Jackson Vereen/FoodPix

Book: All original illustrations created by Totally Incorporated. All other illustrations, on the following pages, are copyright ©1997 by Zedcor, Inc.: 12, 16-17, 19, 22, 25 (lower)-26, 28 (lower), 32-34, 36, 43, 49 (upper)-50, 64, 77, 83-84, 89, 97-98, 106, 112-113, 118 (lower), 123, 133-134, 143-145, 147 (upper), 150, 152-153, 158, 186, 191, 201-202, 206, 212-213, 217, 219, 221-222, 226 (upper)-227, 236, 247, 276-277, 280, 282-286, 298, 305-306, 310-311, 313, 315, 328 (upper), 361.

Art Models: Yoga:Jacqueline Shaffer (principal), Stephanie Henke, Dana Magsumbol, Jim Watson; Acupressure: Elizabeth Moore (principal), Andrew J.S. Somerville; Exercise: Mark Rogers.

Abbreviations

c	in homeopathic dosages, indicating a dilution ratio of 1 part to 99 parts	ml	milliliter
cal	calorie	oz	ounce
F	Fahrenheit	pt	pint
gal	gallon	qt	quart
in	inch	spp.	various species, often used with botanical names of herbs to indicate that more than one species of a plant may be used medicinally
IU	international units, measurement used for fat-soluble vitamins		
lb	pound	tbsp	tablespoon
mcg	microgram	tsp	teaspoon
mg	milligram	x	in homeopathic dosages, indicating a dilution ratio of 1 part to 9 parts

Index

Numerals in italics indicate an illustration of the subject mentioned.

Bursitis: 122, 126

Calluses: 27, 177

Cancer: aflatoxins and: 200, 218; antioxidants and: 12, 278; flavonoids: 12; relieving side effects of treatments for: 215; seven warning signs of: 214. *See also* specific type

Canker sores: preventing: 176, 251, 285; treating: 24, 176, 251, 270

Carpal tunnel syndrome: 130

Cataracts: 42

Celiac disease: 199

Cervical erosion: 323

Cervicitis: 323, 362

Chickenpox: 256, 257, 353; and shingles: 250

Children's health: 346-357; acne: 22, 357; allergies: 351; anorexia: 356, 379, 380; aspirin and: 241, 354; asthma: 158; Attention Deficit Disorder (ADD): 351; bed-wetting: 350, 351; bulimia: 356, 357, 380; chickenpox: 353; colic: 346, 347; coughing: 347, *347;* croup: 282, 347, 348, *348;* dehydration: 349; depression: 354, 355; developmental rate: 346; diaper rash: 257, 349; diarrhea: 349; ear infections: 12; eating disorders: 356, 357, 379, 380; enlarged adenoids: 351; febrile seizures: 348; infants and toddlers: 257, 346, 347, 348, 349, 350, 351; measles: 352; mononucleosis: 220, 354; mumps: 352; Reye's syndrome: 354; roseola: 349; scarlet fever: 354; SIDS: 347; teenagers: 354, 355, 356, 357; teething: 266, 349, 350; thumbsucking: 350

Chlamydia: 330, 360

Cholesterol: 12, 151; HDL ("good"): 11, 12, 152; LDL ("bad"): 12, 151, 152, 154; lowering: 10, 12, 13, 145, 150, 153, 261; test do's and don't's: 151

Cirrhosis: 215, 266

Colds: cause of: 27; flying with: 306, 307; myths about: 27; preventing: 26, 27, 242, 299; treating: 24-27, 240, 241, 257, 260, 270, 282

Cold sores: 176, 251, 285

Colic: 346, 347

Colitis: 193, 194, 282

Colon: 11, 13

Colorectal cancer: fiber and: 11, 13, 280

Congestion: 24, 25, 26; lung: 244, 267; nasal: 117, 118, 159, 168, 169, 241

Conjunctivitis: 110, 260

Constipation: preventing: 13, 43, 197, 281; treating: 43, 197, 256

Contraception: 329, 365, 366

Corns: 177

Coronary artery disease: 147

Coughs: 27, 28, *28,* 214, 241, 259, 267, 347, *347*

Crib death: 347

Crohn's disease: 193

Croup: 282, 347, 348, *348*

Cuts: 229, 230, 231, 232; herbs for: 231, 257, 259, 263, 271, 272

Cystitis: 208, 370

Cysts: 177, 328

Dandruff: 182

Dehydration: 297, 349

Depression: in children: 354, 355; mononucleosis-induced: 220, 354; treating: 74, *74,* 87, 91, *91,* 97, 265, 383, 384, 385, *385,* 386, 387. *See also* Mood enhancers

Diabetes: and chronic impotence: 343; kidney problems and: 201; preventing: 44; symptoms of: 18, 208

Diaper rash: 257, 349

Diarrhea: in infants and children: 349; magnesium supplements and: 107; medication induced: 195, 258; preventing water-and-food-caused while traveling: 312, 313; treating: 191, 195, 314, 315

Diet: antioxidants in: 10, 12, 76, 219, 278; for boosting immune system: 74, 77; fat in: 155, 156, 276, 322, 340;

care of while traveling: 312; cold: 287; corns: 177; exercise to strengthen: 45; plantar warts: 179; varicose veins of: 181
Fertility: body fat and low: 367; impaired in men: 336; impaired in women: 328; smoking-impaired: 366
Fever blisters: *See* Cold sores
Fevers: 257
Fiber: 13, 22, 280, 281, 283
Flavonoids: 12, 147
Flu: preventing: 18, 70; treating: 28, 191, 242, 257, 260, 270. *See also* Stomach flu
Flying: 306, 307, 308, 309
Folliculitis: 249
Food poisoning: 194, 216
Fractures: 235, 264
Free radicals: 46, 74, 278
Frostbite: 231, 234

Gallstones: 194
Gas: causes of: 186, 188, 283; treating: 29, 187, 188, *188,* 258
Gastritis: 191
Gastroenteritis: 191, 245, 282
Gingivitis: 252
Goiter: 265
Gonorrhea: 362, 364, *364*
Gout: preventing: 132, 281; treating: 44, 133, 281
Graves' Disease: treating eye symptoms of: 216
Groin pulls: 131, *131*
Gums: diseases of: 252; maintaining healthy: 12, 44, 45, 267, 270; receding and tooth hypersensitivity: 184

Hair: 45, 183, 264
Hamstrings: 132, *132*
Hands: cold: 287
Hangover: 29, 286
Hay fever: 118; herbal do's and don'ts for: 30; treating: 168, *168,* 282, 285
Headaches: 30-31, 89, 260, 271

Health, whole body: 10-17; back: 136-141; bones: 133-134; digestive system: 186-199; ears: 113-117; eyes: 110-113; hair: 182-183; heart: 142-157; joints: 122-127; kidneys and urinary tract: 200-209; muscles and tendons: 127-132, 135; nails: 185; nose: 118; respiratory system: 158-171; skin: 172-182; teeth: 184; throat: 119-121. *See also* specific ailment; specific topic
Hearing loss: 46, 114, *114,* 115, *115,* 284
Heart: 343; antioxidants and: 10, 278; aspirin and: 13, 148; strengthening: 142, 264; and stress: 157; "target zone" rate during exercise: 292; Vitamin E and: 10, 143. *See also* Heart disease
Heartburn: 32, 190
Heart disease: angina: 142, 144, 146; anxiety-induced palpitations: 62; arrhythmias: 217; atherosclerosis: 146, 147, 276, 343; coronary artery disease: 147; decreasing risk of: 142, 143, 144, 145, 154, 155, 343; diet and prevention: 13, 143, 144, 145, 150, 153, 154, 155, 156, 217; dietary supplements and prevention: 10, 143, 147, 148, 151, 152, 153; exercise and: 148, 292; interpersonal relationships and: 149; pets and: 17; smoking and: 150; stress and: 143; tachycardia: 217; and women: 322. *See also* Cholesterol; Heart
Heat: symptoms of illness caused by: 299
Helicobacter pylori: as cause of ulcers: 192, 246
Hemorrhoids: 88, 277; preventing: 43, 281; treating: 32
Hepatitis: 266
Herbs for healing: 256-273; alfalfa: 256, *256;* aloe: 256, *256;* black cohosh: 256, *256;* boneset: 257, *257;* burdock: 257, *257;* calendula: 257, *257;* cayenne: 258, *258;* chamomile: 258, *258;* chaste tree: 258, *258;* coltsfoot:

Kidneys: acute disease of and wild mushrooms: 201; avoiding problems: 200, 201, 202, 206; cancer of: 200, 202; cause of infections: 247; treatment of infections: 247

Kidney stones: preventing: 206, 207, 277, 284; treating: 205, 206, 207

Laryngitis: 121, 242

Laughter: 18; as mood enhancer: 95, 96, 97

Legs: preventing nightime cramps of: 128; sciatica as cause of pain in: 141; spasms of: 128; ulcers of: 262

Lice: 35

Liver: 11, 47, 266

Liver cancer: 218

Lock jaw: See Tetanus

Lungs: 160, 161, 162, 164. See also Allergies; Congestion; Emphysema

Lupus: 219

Lyme disease: 252

Macular degeneration: 12, 219

Malaria: 305

Manic depression: 219, 385

Measles: 257, 352

Melanoma: checking skin for: 16; and moles: 181; preventing: 16, 180

Menopause: 49; hormone replacement therapy and: 47; hot flashes: 318, 319, 324, 325, 326; relieving symptoms of: 256, 320, 324, 325, 368; sex after: 368

Men's health: 336-357; cronic prostatitis: 340; enlarged prostate: 340; genital warts: 360, 361, 363; hair loss: 342; herpes: 361; impotence: 337, 338, 342, 343, 369; infertility: 336; inguinal hernia: 338, 339; jock itch: 35, 341; premature ejaculation: 338, 369; prostate cancer: 17, 222, 339, 340; prostate inflammation: 49, 271; sexually transmitted disease symptoms. See Sexually transmitted diseases;

shaving: 249, 341; testicular cancer: 336; trama to testicles: 342

Menstruation: 256; breast pain: 321, 331; cramps: 259, 273, 319, 319, 326, 327, 371; heavy: 327; intercourse during: 321; irregularity: 258, 320; onset at puberty: 355; PMS: 258, 277, 320, 321, 331, 332, 371; premenstrual syndrom: 258, 271, 277, 320, 321, 331, 332; tampons and: 318

Mental health: 374-387; alcoholism: 380, 381, 382; anorexia: 356, 379, 380; anxiety. See Anxiety; bulimia: 356, 357, 380; coping skill development: 376, 377, 378; coping strategies: 94-107; depression. See Depression; diagnosis: 377, 378; dysthymia: 383; improving: 19, 374, 375; manic depression: 219, 385; memory: 42; obsessive-compulsive disorder (OCD): 379; organic diseases and: 376, 378; panic: 375, 378; phobias: 377; seasonal affective disorder (SAD): 384; stress. See Stress. See also Mood enhancers

Moles: 16, 181

Moniliasis: 362

Mononucleosis: 220, 260, 354

Mood enhancers: 94-107; exercise: 97, 98, 99, 99; laughter: 18, 95, 96, 97; music: 19; pets: 97; relaxation techniques: 99, 99, 100, 100

Morning sickness: 261, 269, 320, 329

Motion sickness: 36, 261, 308, 309, 309, 310

Multiple sclerosis: 220

Mumps: 352

Muscles: 128-133; cramps of: 36, 297; hamstring stretches: 132, 132; massage for back: 139; preventing nighttime cramps of: 128; reducing stress in neck: 135, 135; relaxant for: 139; spasms in leg: 128; treating sore and injured: 127, 129, 130, 236, 259, 266, 296, 341

Mushrooms: for boosting immune sys-

ing: 174; hives: 34, 177, 179; impetigo: 179; inflammation of: 177, 259, 263, 265; irritations: 256, 257; minor burns: 174, 232, 233, 2331; plantar warts: 179; poison ivy: 37, 175; poison oak: 37, 175; poison sumac: 37, 175; psoriasis: 180, 222, 263, 283; rashes. *See* Rashes; rosacea: 173; ulcers: 257, 259
Skin cancer: and childhood sunburn: 180; moles and: 181; prevention of: 16
Sleep: 83-86, 116; adequate and good health: 10; inducing: 75, 84, 86, 258, 264, 268, 273; insomnia: 62, 84, 86, 271; overstimulation and: 84, 85; resetting internal clock: 83, 310, 311; snoring and: 37, 85
Sleep apnea: 85
Smoking: avoiding as key to good health: 10; and heart disease: 150; and impaired fertility: 366; importance of quitting: 75; and impotence: 337; quitting: 44; and respiratory illnesses: 158; and skin: 15, 44
Sneezing: 37, *37,* 117
Snoring: 37, 85
Sore throat: 38, 119-121, 214, 240, 257, 263, 267, 270
Spanish fly: 371
Splinters: 237
Sprains: 127, 130, 131, 235, 236, 259, 298
Sties: 113
Stomach: aspirin and: 13; revitalizing: 193, *193*
Stomach cancer: 190
Stomach flu: 282. *See also* Gastroenteritis
Strains: 127, 130, 131, 235, 259, 266, 298
Strep throat: 243
Stress: 62; alcohol and: 11; and binge eating: 280; coping strategies for: 19, 54-65, *55, 63;* and heart: 143, 157; and hives: 178; and immune system: 71, 72, 73; pets and: 17; reducing: 72, 73, 271. *See also* Relaxation

Strokes: decreasing risk of: 11, 13, 42, 46, 50, 143, 144, 155; results of: 42
Sudden Infant Death Syndrome (SIDS): 347
Sun: and eyes: 42, 298; and skin cancer: 16
Sunburn: preventing: 180, 181; and skin cancer: 180; treating: 38-39, 180, 181, 231, 256
Sweating: 174, 287
Swimmer's ear: 115, 116

T
chycardia: 217, 376
Tampons: 364
Teenagers' health: 272, 354, 355, 356, 357
Teeth: 184
Teething: 266, 349, 350
Tendinitis: 127, 131
Tendons: 128
Tennis elbow: 129, 237, 297
Testicles: cancer of: 336; injury to: 342
Tetanus: 18, 253, 304
Thumbsucking: 350
Thyroid: exercise to improve function of: 223, *223;* hyperthyroidism (overactive): 376; underactive: 81, 88, 89, 265
Tinnitus: 116, 284
TMJ: 135, 286
Tongue: 229
Toxic shock syndrome: 332
Traveler's diarrhea: 191, 282, 312, 313, 314, 315
Traveling: essentials to take along: 305, 306; health insurance for: 304; immunizations for: 304, 305; jet lag and: 83, 310, 311, 312; maintaining health while: 304-315; medical emergencies during: 315; and motion sickness: 308, 309, 310; reducing stress during: 64; while pregnant: 304
Tremors: 62
Trichomoniasis: 363